talking about sex

talking about sex

Derek C. Polonsky, M.D.

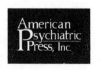

American Psychiatric Press, Inc.

Washington, DC
London, England

Copyright © 1995 Derek C. Polonsky
ALL RIGHTS RESERVED
Manufactured in the United States of America on acid-free paper
98 97 96 95   4 3 2 1
First Edition

American Psychiatric Press, Inc.
1400 K Street, N.W., Washington, DC   20005

Library of Congress Cataloging-in-Publication Data
Polonsky, Derek C., 1945-
    Talking about sex / Derek C. Polonsky.
       p.   cm.
    Includes bibliographical references (p.) and index.
    ISBN 0-88048-719-4
    1. Sex.   2.   Sex (Psychology).   3.   Man-woman relationships.   4.   Communication in sex—United States.   I. Title.
  HQ21.P587   1995
  306.7—dc20   95-37799
  for Library of Congress   CIP

British Library Cataloguing in Publication Data
A CIP record is available from the British Library.

Contents

Introduction

I did not consciously choose to get into the field of sex therapy. Actually, it was the couples I began treating as a young psychiatrist who forced me to confront my ignorance and to develop an awareness of sexual dysfunctions and methods of treatment. Nothing I learned as a student at Harvard Medical School had prepared me for the fact that once my patients began to trust me they might begin talking openly about their sexual problems.

Initially, I avoided any direct discussion with patients about their sexual concerns, unknowingly pretending that this part of their lives did not warrant attention. When couples raised sexual questions, I felt awkward and self-conscious, and at times could feel my face flush with embarrassment. Amazingly, throughout 4 years of training to become a psychiatrist, I'd not had a single lecture devoted solely to sex, and I lacked a basic understanding of sexual physiology and functioning. I firmly believed the traditional psychiatric school of thought, which held that all sexual difficulties were expressions of deep-seated psychological conflicts that had to be identified and understood before any improvement could be expected. The idea of suggesting to people what to do in their sexual lives went against all I had learned in my training. I had been taught to reflect and understand; giving directions was frowned upon. There were times when I felt that I was barely keeping ahead of my patients' questions by reading Masters and Johnson's work and Helen Singer Kaplan's *The New Sex Therapy.*

I've come to realize that the almost unlimited range of possible human sexual behavior can confuse any person, regardless of his or her emotional health. Health providers still don't have enough instruction regarding sex, although this is beginning to change. From the stories I hear, I realize that even in our so-called sexually liberated society, many people remain miserable and many relationships suffer because of misconceptions about what is "normal" sexually. Most adults remain too embarrassed to ask their physicians even basic questions.

When couples began telling me that they had sexual problems, not only did I lack information, I also had no experience in having open, adult-to-adult discussions about sex. It did not help that I was much younger than many of the couples I saw as clients, and it felt as if I were asking my parents' friends to elaborate what they did in the bedroom. And yet the more I learned, and the more I talked with my patients, the easier it became. I began to notice that my comfort and competence changed the way my patients could talk about their sexual lives. My office became a safe place where openness was encouraged, information was made available in a frank, nonjudgmental way, and we could laugh and joke while we solved problems. I have witnessed the powerful effects that such openness can have on patients' perceptions of their problems, and have watched dramatic transformations take place as couples have been able to use newly learned skills to open fresh possibilities in their relationships.

Although this book is not directed at children, it does provide information in one place so that parents have a resource to help them communicate about sex. As difficult as it may be, parents need to find ways to explain how bodies develop and babies are born. Like it or not, they provide their children with the models for personal values about physical intimacy. Most important, adults have to be certain that the adolescents in their care know how to keep themselves safe from acquired immunodeficiency syndrome (AIDS) and other sexually transmitted diseases.

Learning to communicate openly about sex early in life can greatly reduce conflicts later—or, better still, prevent them from developing. I remember my own curiosity about sex as an adolescent and having nowhere to turn for information. As a teenager, I never had an open discussion with any adult about sex, and I certainly couldn't imagine couples having conversations in which sexual wishes were explicitly expressed. There was simply no model for this. Discussions with friends were limited because we were all unsure and ignorant and were reluctant to reveal the true extent of our inexperience.

There have been many books published, both professional and popular, covering every aspect of sexual behavior, variety, and expression. Rather than duplicate what others have already done well, I have chosen to refer to those texts I have found particularly useful. There is no one ideal book: some have great illustrations; some are loaded with information; some are oriented toward self-help. This book focuses on talking about sex. It reflects conversations I have had about sex, either directly in my clinical work or through a monthly column I wrote for many years in *FIRST* magazine. The questions asked provide a look at the range of concerns people have. The answers are intended to educate and to reassure. No magical cures are offered, and there are no exhortations to attain Olympian sexual mastery. Instead, what is presented is a frank, open discussion about people's sexual lives.

Acknowledgments

I wish to thank Dr. Carol Nadelson not only for guiding me toward treating couples but also for her advice, support, and encouragement as I learned and integrated the principles of the sexual therapies into my work.

My gratitude also goes to my many patients, whose struggles inspired this book. Listening to their stories has been a unique experience and a special privilege. They have revealed their most intimate thoughts and actions and have entrusted me with their confidences. Through these relationships, I have learned that talking about sex in a straightforward way is powerful and healing. It is from my patients, also, that I learned never to assume anything about sex and always to be open-minded and humble in my formulations.

I am additionally indebted to the readers of *FIRST* magazine, whose frank questions about their sexual concerns provided the impetus to write this book, and to the many people who provided editorial assistance during the 5 years I wrote the column. I owe special thanks to Nuna Albert, who helped structure and organize the questions.

Finally, I want to thank my wife Cathie and my two daughters Sasha and Rachel for being there throughout this endeavor. It is from them that I have learned the most about love and relationships.

*C*hapter 1

Am I Normal?

Am I normal? Is it okay to think like this? What do other people do? Am I the only one who . . . ? Is my body okay? Are my breasts too large? Are they too small? Is my penis big enough? Is the color okay? Do I come too soon? Do I turn him on? Why does it hurt? How do I let him know that what he does doesn't feel good? Can I say no? How do I know if she comes? I don't really feel like it—what's wrong?

Questions, questions. People are interested in and curious about sex—what they do, think, and feel and what others do, think, and feel. Magazines, books, videotapes, and now the Internet are all sources of information about sex that people are seeking out in huge numbers. Surveys about what goes on in the bedroom abound, and they are devoured, studied, and talked about. It wasn't always this way: 20 years ago, the sources of information about sex were very limited.

We are schooled endlessly in almost every aspect of life. We are tested, graded, evaluated, and coached. We are trained and certified. We take exams and get licensed. We are forced into taking continuing education to make sure we keep abreast of trends in our work. We are reexamined and recertified. Yet sex seems to be one huge arena where we are thrown into the ring blind, unprepared, and untrained, with little encouragement to ask questions and with

1

many assumptions that "everyone else knows what to do" and that, if we don't, it is conclusive proof that we have no chance of getting a foothold on the sexual revolution (such as it is) that is alleged to have gripped this nation. Given the resistance to sex education in the schools, rampant teenage pregnancy, the refusal to encourage advertisements for condoms, and the difficulty most of us have in talking to our own kids about the issue, it is no wonder that so many are confused when it comes to sex.

While many seem to master the challenges of being sexual without difficulty, between 20% and 50% of sexually active individuals have trouble with sex at some point in their lives. That translates into roughly 75 million people!

What Is Good Sex?

To be frank, I hate this question. I believe that concerns about how to be "the best" or how to "drive your man (or woman) wild in bed" only add to people's worries about performance and shift the focus away from deriving pleasure. I have done an informal survey of cover articles of women's and men's magazines and have found that it is rare that an issue appears without a cover line screaming out some better way to make love. However, because I am asked this question so often, I have tried in this book to describe some of the ingredients that contribute to enjoyable sex.

In its best form, a long-term relationship with another individual has much to offer: companionship, friendship, support, sharing, and sexual and physical intimacy. I like working with couples because of the potential their relationship has. With couples there are two involved adults who have had different life experiences and who have the capacity for putting ideas, wishes, and feelings into words. There is an opportunity to have an impact on the other person; it is possible to let that person know what one's needs are, to discuss ways in which one might feel hurt and vulnerable, and to derive support and caring from each other.

Helping couples tap into that potential is both challenging and rewarding. Couples' relationships are intense and fluid; nothing remains fixed, and change is constant. The different dynamics and influences affecting couples are unlimited. There may be external changes and stress (jobs, relatives, finances); there may be internal torment (self-esteem, depression, anger, loss). The interpersonal forces may be complementary or may be misaligned, and there are always unpredictable and uncontrollable life events. Throughout the fabric of a relationship are woven sexual and physical expressions, which shift and change over time.

Six Components of a Good Sex Life

Sexual feelings are unlike any others; there is a special charge that comes with physical tension associated with heightened arousal. To share and express these feelings with another individual offers the possibility of an intensely pleasurable encounter or a painfully devastating one. A common view is that feelings should be instinctive and natural, and in many instances they are. However, the complexity of interpersonal experiences between humans changes that. For many, letting go sexually and exposing that intimate side requires a solid base of trust and a willingness to tolerate vulnerability.

What are the components of a satisfying and exciting sexual life?

1. *Being able to talk openly with each other about sexual feelings without fear of disapproval or rejection.* This talk might cover what you like, what feels good, and what does not. It's important to recognize and reconcile differences about sexual preferences, to learn to be honest without being hurtful, and to negotiate compromise. Being direct and open is key to becoming attuned to each other's sexual rhythms. Despite what is shown in the movies, most of us cannot read minds, and we do

not have built-in radar to let us know what our partner's experience is like.

2. *An atmosphere of mutual trust and respect.* I know this seems hackneyed, but for most people it is crucial to feel that the person they are with will not intentionally cause them emotional pain. A climate in which you can feel safe will promote more openness than one in which you feel on guard. You need to know that limits will be respected, uncertainties will not be challenged, and your partner will reciprocate. Almost everyone experiences uncertainty and lapses of confidence in day-to-day life, and sex is no exception. Given the nature of the sexual experience, these feelings are all the more intense. If two people feel safe with each other, they will be freer to explore a wider range of activities and be open to more adventure.

3. *A willingness to take risks.* We are not talking about skydiving or shooting the rapids! This risk-taking involves letting your partner in on some thoughts that have remained hidden, a particular curiosity, a wish to try something, a thought that may sound "weird." In other words, this is self-exposure—sharing private feelings, dreams, and worries—and it requires courage. Being more assertive about sexual needs, while easy for some, does not come naturally for many people.

4. *Knowledge.* Despite the increased availability of sexual information, many people are woefully ignorant sexually. Knowledge opens doors to understanding and growth. The more people understand about how humans work sexually, what happens, and how things sometimes *don't* work right, the greater their ability to make changes that can enhance satisfaction for themselves and for their partners. In many instances, some basic information and advice for overcoming the roadblocks that inevitably occur in any long-term relationship can be liberating. There are many excellent and useful resources available that offer this knowledge, and you'll find some listed in the appendix ("Information Resources") at the back of this book.

5. *Humor.* I know that you cannot "mandate" humor, but it makes such a difference to be able to laugh and have fun. Kidding around and being playful are enjoyable and allow for more spontaneity and less worry about performance. All too often I hear couples describing a dramatic transformation taking place as they cross the threshold of the bedroom: suddenly things get serious and performance tension rises.

6. *Physical fitness.* I have admired and secretly envied people who exercise often without effort. To be honest, I wish I could pay someone to exercise for me! Nevertheless, regular exercise is important and contributes to a general sense of well-being. Being in reasonable physical shape helps people feel good about their bodies and is one of the many variables that can affect your sexual and sensual state. I should emphasize that good sex and how you feel about someone are not determined by great looks or physical perfection. Judging from movie portrayals of couples having sex, this activity is reserved for the fit and the beautiful. Nothing could be further from the truth!

Sexual Behavior: Common Misperceptions

In 1948, Alfred Kinsey published his ground-breaking study of sexual practices, *Sexual Behavior of the Human Male*, to be forever known as "The Kinsey Report." This was the first time that a large number of people were asked questions about their sexual activities. The report shattered myths about abstinence, masturbation, age at first intercourse, and frequencies of sexual activities. Needless to say, it also made many people uncomfortable!

Kinsey brought curiosity about what people do out into the open. This process has continued with ever-increasing studies, interviews, articles, and discussions about sexual behavior. I think the usefulness of these writings is in describing the enormous range and variety of sexual interests and activities. What is missing, however, is a recognition that people are different and that each individual may choose a sexual style that is unique to him or her. I have seen many couples who have an enjoyable and satisfying time together sexually, but who read one of the surveys that states that "couples have intercourse 2.3 times per week," or something like that, and wonder whether there is something wrong with them because their pattern is different. The questions and answers that form the body of this book deal with these differences and preferences. Rather than conforming to what the statisticians say is "usual," I encourage people to explore what feels welcome, enjoyable, and exciting to them.

Through listening to couples' concerns, I've noticed that certain misperceptions repeatedly come up. Briefly, these center on the following topics:

* **Interest and curiosity about sex:** It is striking how often people think that they are somehow abnormal if they want specific information about sex. Buying books about sex feels awkward, and there is almost the wish that such books would come in brown covers! Magazines such as *Playboy* and *Penthouse* cater to a desire people have to look and see. Gratifying this wish is like an adult version of playing "doctor," where "I'll show you mine if you show me yours." I feel that much of the X-rated video industry similarly caters to this curiosity factor. People wonder, "What do others do? What do they look like?" and feel some excitement in watching. I believe that the sadomasochism that has gained so much attention *is* problematic. Although I don't think that the books or videos *cause* this behavior, I do consider it to be a reflection of a very troubled view of relationships.

* **Masturbation:** It is still surprising the strong feelings that masturbation elicits in people. We have come a long way from really believing that it leads to insanity, but the very mixed feelings (often negative) with which the subject is approached are truly remarkable—and quite a burden for people. The fact is, roughly 90% of teenage boys and about 75% of teenage girls

masturbate. It is an activity that is associated with pleasure and leads to knowing something about one's sexual feelings and responses. By discovering and enjoying the feelings from one's body, the foundations of seeing sex as something to feel good about and to be shared are laid down. Masturbation continues throughout life—and 45%–50% of adults admit to continuing this practice with no demonstrable mental deterioration! In fact, masturbation may enhance a good sexual relationship.

* **Oral sex:** Fellatio (sucking a penis; also known as a *blow job*) and cunnilingus (licking and sucking the clitoris and vaginal lips; also know as *going down on*) are extremely common. Roughly 75%–80% of people engage in these activities. Like masturbation, the topic of oral sex is also associated with a great deal of negative feelings, disgust being the most common. The reasons for this are complicated—some of the questions and answers will deal with these concerns (e.g., see page 85).

* **Anal sex:** I must admit I was surprised when discovering that roughly 25% of married couples engage in anal intercourse—despite repeatedly telling myself that I should never make assumptions about what people do! Among the teenage population, anal intercourse has become more popular because there is the belief that this means "I haven't really done it" and also you can't get pregnant that way.

* **Bondage and variations:** The whole range of activities that include handcuffs, leather, and tying people up has gained more publicity recently. There is a spectrum ranging from playful experimentation to behavior that is quite dangerous. Although the publicity has been sensational, the number of people who engage in these activities is quite small in terms of percentages.

Common Sexual Problems

Sex is a private and very intense part of people's lives. The ability to function sexually is often taken for granted, yet it can be disrupted very easily, with painful consequences for the couple whose sexual relationship is impaired. Serious sexual difficulties affect from 30% to 50% of couples. What adds to the emotional suffering are the difficulties couples have in talking openly about sexual problems and the fear that not much can be done. Millions of people carry with them a sense of shame, embarrassment, failure, disappointment, and sadness because they believe their sexual abilities are deficient—often with the powerful conviction that no one else has any difficulties. For this reason, I want to spell out clearly what are common sexual problems (the technical word is *dysfunction*) and how they can be treated.

Sexual Problems Affecting Women

Sexual problem	How common	Description
No arousal	10%–15%	• A mental block prevents woman from getting turned on. • Anxiety is usually a factor. • Because vaginal lubrication does not occur, intercourse is uncomfortable or painful.
Orgasm difficulties	15%–20%	• Woman has never had an orgasm. Woman can have an orgasm with masturbation but not with partner.
No orgasm with intercourse	40%	• This condition is *not* an indication of a problem. Great variability exists in the amount and type of stimulation women need to climax. For many, the kind of stimulation they receive during intercourse, while pleasurable, does not provide enough clitoral stimulation for orgasm. Some direct stimulation,

whether provided by self or by partner, can make the difference.

Pain with intercourse 5%

- Pain can be caused by a vaginal infection. When the infection is treated, the pain goes away.
- *Vulvar vestibulitis* is a condition associated with intense pain that can be localized in a particular area of the vagina. Many women with this condition have suffered enormously and have even been labeled "neurotic" because the proper diagnosis was not made. Treatment is slow, using a variety of medications designed to decrease inflammation and increase muscular relaxation.
- *Vaginismus* is a condition in which there may be such intense pain that the muscles around the vagina go into spasm and intercourse is *impossible*. Many couples exist who have been married for years but have never been able to have intercourse because of this problem. Treatment involves diagnosis and then careful coaching using vaginal dilators.

Inhibited sexual desire 30%

- In this condition, the "machinery" works fine and the woman can be fully responsive. The trouble is that the interest is simply not present. Causes are complicated; see pages 65–68.

Sexual Problems Affecting Men

Sexual problem	How common	Description
Erectile difficulties	10%	• Inability to get or to maintain an erection. The cause may be psychological (e.g., worry about performance, low self- esteem, fear of intimacy) or physical (e.g., a medical condition that can be treated; see pages 34–37). Once started, however, the cycle is reinforced, because failure becomes anticipated and repeated.
Orgasm difficulties	25%	• *Premature ejaculation:* Orgasm cannot be controlled; man comes very quickly. This condition is very frustrating for both partners. Anxiety only makes the problem worse; it can become the dominating focus of the sexual relationship. Most cases of premature ejaculation can be easily treated with a variety of behavioral techniques and trials of medications.
		• *Retarded ejaculation:* Man cannot come with a partner. Causes are complicated; condition may respond to simple behavioral suggestions or may require a combination of individual and couple approaches.
		• *Painful ejaculation:* Usually indicates an infection of the prostate gland that needs antibiotic treatment.
Inhibited sexual desire	30%	• Ability to perform is intact, but there is profound lack of interest. Causes are complicated; see pages 65–68.

*C*hapter 2

User's Guide to Sexual Responses

*I*n the mid-1950s, a gynecologist, Dr. William Masters, and his associate, Virginia Johnson, a nurse, studied human sexual responses directly for the first time. They looked at how people reacted to sexual stimulation and learned much about responses in both men and women. They examined the changes that occur in the sex organs, the adjustment to blood flow and breathing, and discovered what happens to our bodies as we become more turned on. They also saw how the smooth operation could be interrupted and how drastically sexual function could be affected by many things. Their work produced a much clearer understanding of the physiological process of sexual arousal and response. In addition, for the first time, a treatment was available that addressed specific disorders and did not require that people have in-depth therapy to bring about changes in their sexual functioning.

Before Masters and Johnson, we had two words to describe sexual difficulties: *frigid* and *impotent*—terms that sounded more like a jail sentence than a diagnosis. Through the work of these researchers, we now have a much better appreciation of what affects sexual responses and how this happens.

Sex Is Complicated

The longer I study human sexuality, the more I realize that sex is complicated, variable, and elusive and cannot be packaged into a neat formula. For some, sex is a trial to be endured; for others, it seems to be effortless; and for most, there are times when sex is great and times when sex is terrible. Sex can be exciting simply because it feels good and is a source of physical pleasure; sex can also be a vehicle through which two people express emotional closeness. Some find sexual feelings strange and unwelcome, and some shy away from intimacy.

For an individual who is insecure about himself or herself, sex with someone who is also unsure can be awful, with each reinforcing the anxiety and discomfort in the other. That same insecure person, however, can be very different if his or her partner is comfortable with sex and enjoys it. People can function very differently with different partners. Being with someone who is relaxed and open can help the "uptight" partner feel more at ease and facilitate the enjoyment of sex.

For most couples, sex varies over the course of the relationship. It is tantalizing when the relationship is new, comfortable as the couple becomes more committed, and often problem-filled as a couple settles into a long-term relationship. Couples are frequently puzzled by this paradox. As they become more settled into a family life with each other, they begin to see and experience in their partner characteristics they saw in various members of their original family, and this may affect the sexual relationship. If one partner comes from a family that was very critical, that person may misperceive cues as critical when no criticism was intended, and sexual pleasure may diminish as a result.

Many people feel that sex is great only in the context of a caring, loving relationship where commitment is established. For others, sex may be great only where there is no commitment and where they know little about each other's inner lives. As soon as they get to know their partners better, sexual interest wanes.

As if all these confusing emotional issues around sex were not enough, there are the physical aspects to contend with. Human sexual feelings and interactions are extremely complex, and our physiological responses are no less so.

Human Sexual Functioning

It is startling how much people do not know about their sexual responses and how their bodies work. Having a user's manual can be quite helpful at times.

Female Sexual Response

Using volunteer subjects, Masters and Johnson studied sexual responses in their lab. They were clearly surprised at the willingness of their subjects to engage in a variety of sexual activities that allowed them to take careful note of what was happening all over their bodies. These responses usually begin with sexually arousing thoughts that result in feeling "turned on." This feeling becomes more intense when the activities involve a partner.

The first thing that happens for a woman is a tingling in the clitoris and vagina and the production of lubrication in the vaginal lining. As sexual activity continues, the vagina increases in length and the nerves in the genital area are further stimulated, resulting in the woman's feeling sexually excited. The heart begins to beat more rapidly, blood pressure goes up, and the rate of breathing increases. An orgasm may occur, a rush of intense, almost indescribable feeling in the pelvic area with strong, enjoyable contractions of the pelvic muscles. Following an orgasm, some women have a second or third or more, while others feel a deep sense of relaxation and pleasure. During this time, blood pressure and breathing return to their normal levels, and the genitals return to their prearousal state.

Sensations and Sensitivity

There is a huge collection of nerve endings in the clitoris. Direct stimulation of the clitoris is a personal thing: for some women it feels great; for others, more indirect stimulation by rubbing the area around the clitoris is preferable. The *labia*, or vaginal lips, are also sensitive to touch, and the outer part of the vagina contains nerves that result in pleasurable feelings. The inner two-thirds of the vagina does not have many nerve endings and is not a source of much sensation.

Steps to Orgasm

* **Interest and desire:** These feelings are initiated in the brain and function like the starter for an engine; they get things going. Attraction and "chemistry" are crucial. Personal and interpersonal issues can have powerful effects on this "start-up" mechanism.
* **Tingling sensations in sexual organs:** The woman feels increased tingling and sensitivity in the genitals. The vagina lengthens and the clitoris becomes enlarged.
* **Lubrication produced in vagina:** With increasing arousal, lubrication is produced by the vaginal walls, resulting in feelings of moistness. There is continuous feedback to the brain that either reinforces the feelings or inhibits the responses.
* **Heart rate and breathing increase**
* **Sexual feelings continue to build**
* Orgasm occurs: There is a range of different responses for women; some women are able to have an orgasm easily with a variety of sexual activities. Others require some specific attention; this may include particular attention during foreplay or more direct stimulation of the genitals (clitoris or vagina). This may be done with the partner's hand or fingers or may involve oral sex, using the lips or tongue. Some women do not reach orgasm through intercourse alone; others do. Some women have several orgasms; others do not. The important point is that everyone is different. You need to learn what arouses you and how your body responds to particular forms of stimulation.
* **Relaxation follows**

Male Sexual Response

The emotional responses in the man are similar to those in the woman. There is interest and desire, followed by physical changes associated with feeling sexually turned on. The first reaction is that the penis gets hard. The mechanism is complicated, though the principle is simple. Usually blood flows in and out of the penis, much like water flowing through a garden hose. When a man begins to get aroused, the brain sends a message that shuts off a series of valves in the blood vessels of the penis so that blood continues to flow in but cannot flow out.

If you were to shut off the flow at the end of a garden hose, the hose would become firmer as water was pumped in. This is just what happens with the penis. Other changes include an increase in the heart rate, increased blood pressure, and more rapid breathing. The man feels aroused, and as sexual activity continues, feeling in the penis intensifies. Most of the nerves carrying sensation to the penis are concentrated in the head of the penis (or *glans*). After a while, the sensations become very intense and result in an orgasm (the intense feeling) and ejaculation (the shooting out of semen from the tip of the penis). A feeling of relaxation follows, and the penis is no longer erect. There is a period when another erection and orgasm will not occur because the body requires some "recharging." This is called the *refractory period*. It may only be a few minutes in a teenager and may be several hours for a man in his mid-50s.

Sensations and Sensitivity
Direct stimulation of the head of the penis may feel very exciting, but (as with the clitoris) the intensity may become uncomfortable. The shaft is less sensitive, and the skin around the penis shaft is loose and movable. The *scrotum* (the sac that contains the testicles) is similar to the labia in being sensitive to light touch. Fondling the testicles may feel good, although too much pressure can cause pain.

Steps to Orgasm

*   **Interest and desire:** As with women, it is the brain, the organ that mediates complex feelings, that is the source of the unique experience we identify as sexual desire. Feeling in the penis increases and the man feels turned on.
*   **Penis becomes erect:** There is a building sensation of fullness, and arousal builds. Blood flows into the penis, "valves" shut, and the penis enlarges and becomes hard.
*   **Increase in blood pressure and rate of breathing:** Erection and full arousal are *not* the same thing. Men require time to become fully aroused psychologically and physiologically. They usually need more direct touching with increasing age.
*   **Orgasm and ejaculation:** This includes an intense feeling, with waves of muscular contraction with ejaculation. With infrequent sexual activity, men may ejaculate quite soon. For many men, control may be difficult, and they may ejaculate before they want to. This is known as premature ejaculation.
*   **Resolution:** Sex organs return to prearousal state.
*   **Refractory period:** Men need time to "recover" before they can have another erection and orgasm. This time increases with age. The refractory period may last a few minutes for teenagers and several hours for older men.

Sexual Downers:
Things That Cause Problems

Controversy exists as to the percentage of "medical" versus "psychological" causes of sexual difficulties. It depends on whom you listen to. The important point is that a thorough evaluation involves paying attention to both medical and psychological issues.

Clearly, in the past, we may have erred on the side of assuming too readily that a sexual problem had a psychological cause. Our understanding of sexual physiology continues to grow and so does our appreciation of the medical factors responsible for sexual dysfunction.

Here's a rough guide of possible medical and physical causes of sexual problems, plus personal and relationship issues that may affect sexual behavior.

Physical Issues

Medications: Many medications may affect sexual functioning. If you take a medication and notice a change, discuss it with your doctor.

Illnesses:
Alcoholism
Arthritis
Diabetes
Disease of blood vessels
Heart disease
Heavy smoking (emphysema)
High blood pressure
Multiple sclerosis
Pituitary gland disorders
Spinal cord injuries
Surgery (including prostate surgery, hysterectomy, mastectomy, and colon surgery)
Thyroid disorders

Personal Issues

Anxiety
Lack of confidence
Lack of self-esteem/poor body image
Performance worries
Inhibitions
Lack of information
Religious conflicts
Childhood sexual abuse

Other emotional issues
Depression
Work conflicts

Relationship Issues

Jealousy
√ Avoidance of closeness
Competition
Difficulty with anger
Fear of criticism
Outside pressures

Chapter 3

Now—Let's Talk!

I struggled over the title of this book. Friends and colleagues thought I needed something zippy, a title that would catch the potential reader's attention. "Okay," I said, "what would you recommend?" There followed many suggestions, like "Sex Talk," "The Ins and Outs of Sex," "Dr. Derek Talks . . . ." I kept coming back to what I did in my office—helping my patients *talk about sex*. I know that there is more information about sex readily available today than ever before, and yet having the information does not change things for many couples who have problems. What often *does* help is **talking about sex** in a safe place, with a supportive, encouraging adult.

A recurrent theme I notice as I listen to couples is that people don't talk much about their sexual thoughts, wishes, and worries. Particularly their worries. Oh, there is a lot of innuendo, and of course many sexually colored jokes. We often have opportunities to discuss these issues indirectly when the sexual indiscretions of politicians or celebrities make the news. But for most people, acquiring knowledge about sex is a haphazard, catch-as-catch-can affair.

I often tell the joke about the boy who asked his mother, "Where did I come from?"

She thought for a moment and then said, "We got you at Bloomingdale's."

"Well, where did you come from?" he continued.

"They found me in the cabbage patch," was her next answer, offered with a straight face.

"What about Grandma?" he persisted.

"Oh, that's easy—the stork brought her!"

The next day, the boy went to school and handed in his composition, in which he had written, "The reason I am so complex is that my family has not had normal sexual relations for three generations!"

Although the evasiveness demonstrated by this parent is extreme to the point of silliness, the story illustrates a very real point: most people do not find it easy to talk or share ideas about sex. I have repeatedly thought about the absence of role models in this process. In all the years I have been asking, I probably have encountered only a handful of people whose parents had open, direct conversations with them about sexuality that were helpful and guiding. I recall a time, when I was still in training to become a psychiatrist, in which the designated speaker for a lecture failed to show, and one of the staff psychiatrists presented a case study of a couple with a sexual problem. The embarrassment amongst this group of mental health professionals as sexual material was discussed was truly amazing. It should have come as no surprise. There was little teaching regarding sex and again no role models for talking about the subject openly and comfortably.

I almost always preface a meeting with my patients by saying, "Look, I know it feels odd to be discussing your most intimate thoughts and experiences with a perfect stranger. I will try and make this comfortable, and I am sure you will find that it gets easier." And it invariably does. There are times when I am surprised at the frankness of the discussions that take place in my office. Within one or two meetings, the barriers to talking melt away.

The indirectness with which people refer to body parts and activities mirrors our culture's discomfort with these topics. Whenever someone uses words such as "he/she touches me . . . ," I report specifically what I believe they are referring to ("So when he touches your clitoris . . ."—or "when she touches your penis . . . "), thereby providing a model that directness can lead to openness.

I cannot remember any occasion where someone told me that my asking them about their sexual activity was offensive and unwelcome. The opposite is much more common. I was talking with a 20-year-old about his current relationship. We had in the past talked about his sexual experiences, and I knew what kinds of things he struggled with. After he skillfully avoided mentioning anything to do with his and his girlfriend's sexual activities, I asked, "So how have things been sexually?" He smiled, sat back in the chair, and said, "I was waiting for you to ask!"—and then reflected on how much he welcomed knowing that he could talk about his thoughts and observations with me.

In this chapter, I have included a number of questions that come up frequently in my practice. They reflect common worries and concerns that people often have but seldom feel comfortable discussing or seeking information and reassurance about. With almost any other kind of problem in life, resources for help and guidance are readily available and people are often encouraged to pursue them. With concerns about sexuality, however, the silence is thunderous, and often the message is "don't tell and don't ask." Yet whenever people are helped or encouraged to be open, myths are dispelled, information is shared, people feel less alone, and there is a sense of relief.

This chapter starts the conversation about what people do and what problems they face. We'll discuss the topics listed below:

* Inability to have intercourse because the penis cannot be inserted
* Difficulty in consummating a relationship
* Low sexual desire: causes and treatment
* Physical abuse and lack of desire
* Alcoholism and lack of desire
* Man's inability to have orgasm during intercourse
* Trouble delaying ejaculation
* Behavioral therapy for premature ejaculation
* Bereavement and impotence

* Anger and erection problems
* Prevalence and physical causes of impotence
* Diabetes and erection difficulties
* Treatment for physical problems with erection

> **Please help! My husband and I have been married for 5 years and have never been able to have intercourse. Whenever we try, my vagina is so tight that it is impossible for him to put his penis in.**

It appears that you have a condition known as *vaginismus*—an involuntary vaginal spasm or contraction that makes inserting any object, including a penis, very painful and often impossible.

We simply do not understand why this happens, although it generally is viewed as an emotional condition caused by deep-rooted fears about sex. Vaginismus can occur in varying degrees; a related condition, called *apareunia*, is diagnosed when a woman can insert fingers or a tampon but not a penis into her vagina.

What you describe is primary vaginismus. You appear never to have been able to tolerate penetration in any sexual relationship. Another type, secondary vaginismus, flares up suddenly in women who previously enjoyed intercourse. Its onset usually is linked to an emotional trauma, often sexual in nature, but not necessarily so. Secondary vaginismus also can be a reaction to vaginal pain related to an infection, a hormonal imbalance, or physical injury caused by childbirth. A cycle develops in which the woman anticipates pain, which causes an involuntary constriction of the vagina.

Vaginal dilators (insertable objects of graduated sizes to train the muscles to relax) and psychotherapy are the primary treatments for this condition. But many women also benefit from practicing mental relaxation techniques, such as meditation, and from learning more about their sexual anatomy and the physiology of sexual responses. With support and encouragement from a partner, this condition usually can be improved quite quickly.

In the least severe cases, self-help measures sometimes work. Using a mirror, spend some time exploring your vulva and vaginal entrance. That may be all you can do the first session. When you are ready, place some lubricant—such as K-Y Jelly, Astroglide, or another "personal lubricant" (avoid Vaseline or other oil-based formulations)— on a fingertip and gently try to insert it into your vagina. Go slowly and stop at the first sign of a contraction. Wait, then try again. Continue over several days or weeks until you can insert two or three fingers at once. (See the "Self-Help" section in Chapter 7, pages 91–93.)

> In 5 years of marriage, my husband and I have never made love. When we were dating, I thought his reluctance was endearing. I, too, wanted to wait until after the wedding. But now I'm sure there is something wrong. I keep waiting for him to lead the way, but he's even more reluctant to talk about this than I am. He doesn't even want me to see him without his clothes on. I do love him and he says he loves me. Why can't we have a normal life?

Unconsummated marriages are not as rare as you might think. In such situations, the couple often enters into a silent agreement to avoid the discomfort one or both associate with being sexual. Although it suits their emotional needs on one level, the pact also creates a humiliating secret.

It was once thought that the best way to deal with the problem was to help both people understand the underlying conflicts blocking their enjoyment of sex. I've found, however, that it's often better to work on changing behavior. Once a sexual relationship is in place, the psychological underpinnings can be studied. The structure and safety of therapy sessions are enormously reassuring and help each person recognize how he or she feels now.

Obviously, your unconsummated marriage is a problem you can't tackle alone. My best advice is to see a sex therapist. Be sure you find someone who can lead you through the following steps:

* Talking exercises to help you and your husband feel a sense of control, security, and then enjoyment.

❋ Touching exercises with your clothes on to let you simply ex-
   amine what each sensation makes you feel. Gradually, you'll
   begin touching—at first with some clothes off, then, perhaps
   in the dark with all of them removed.
❋ Genital contact without any expectation of arousal. This can
   be a difficult stage; one or both of you may become anxious
   and angry. However, the support of weekly therapy sessions
   should help you to sort out the emotions.

This is the usual way a treatment program is constructed. The
time frame is impossible to predict. I have seen some couples make
rapid gains within a matter of weeks, with absolutely dramatic changes
in their self-esteem; others may take longer and require a combination
of the behavioral exercises and a more traditional therapy.

What causes low sexual desire, and what can be done for someone with this condition?

The causes of inhibited sexual desire are diverse. The condition
may be a reflection of life changes, medications or illness, internal
emotional struggles, or troubled relationships in which the low desire mirrors the emptiness or tension of the marriage (see the
sections on "Inhibited Sexual Desire" and "Low Sexual Desire
and Erectile Difficulties" in Chapter 8, pages 104–105 and 115–
119). Compared with the approach developed by Masters and
Johnson to treat sexual "dysfunctions," treatment of inhibited sexual desire is usually lengthy and change is quite slow. It is common
for therapy to combine several different approaches, using techniques that may require both meeting with each partner individu-
ally and meeting with both partners together. The therapist may
make specific behavioral suggestions (originally developed by Masters and Johnson) and incorporate these into the work of trying to
understand and change the block to sexual pleasure.

My ex-husband hit me. It hasn't been that long since I left him and I'm trying to get my life on track. But I can't seem

to enjoy the company of men. I have no desire, none, for sex. In fact, the thought enrages me.

I would urge you to get counseling to help you recover from your experiences. Women who are victims of domestic violence may mistakenly feel that they have either invited the abuse or deserved it. It is extremely important to know that hitting a partner is *never* acceptable behavior. It would surprise me if you *did* feel like having sex at this point. Right now it probably doesn't feel safe to trust a man or to put yourself in a vulnerable position. Rather than focusing your attention on sex, I would strongly encourage you to first make sure you understand your feelings about what happened during your marriage. Sometimes people find themselves drawn to people who don't treat them well, and you have an opportunity to make sure that you don't repeat a pattern of getting into a relationship with someone whose anger gets out of control.

For 2 years I have had absolutely no sexual desire. During this time, my husband changed jobs and began drinking to the point that I worry he is an alcoholic. Can there be a connection between my depressed sexual interest and his drinking?

Absolutely! Your husband's alcoholism is a loud, clear statement that things are not going well for him, and you are affected by that announcement. This is a warning signal of dramatic changes to come. If you ask your husband, he may deny strenuously that he has a problem, and many people who don't know him as well as you do may agree. It is not surprising that you have less interest in sex. In a sense, your husband has become a stranger, and his behavior probably makes you feel less secure and safe, too.

There is no delicate way of dealing with this. You should contact Al-Anon, a group support system for families of alcoholics. They will offer you extensive guidance as you seek ways to help your husband and yourself. From witnessing several unsuccessful treatments involving alcohol abuse, I've come to realize that no relational change can or will occur unless the drinking (and accompanying depression) is addressed. Once your husband is able to take ownership of that part of his life, there is a good chance that you will be able to heal the relationship.

> **My husband is unable to have an orgasm during intercourse, and I can't help feeling that I'm doing something wrong. Am I?**

Your worry that you are doing something wrong is an all too frequent response. If a partner doesn't have an orgasm or an erection or has some other problem, the refrain becomes "It must be me!" There are many situations that have nothing to do with the partner. It is the unfortunate conspiracy of silence that makes it difficult for couples to share their ideas about what is going on: It would greatly relieve most people to have their partner tell them, "It's not you, there isn't someone else—and frankly the problem existed before we got together."

As to the issue at hand—some men suffer from a condition known as *retarded ejaculation*, in which they can't have an orgasm during intercourse. There is no single cause for this. Sometimes medications inhibit the orgasm reflex (Prozac is one of the better known). In these situations, stopping the drug—if possible—usually solves the problem.

For many men, concerns about losing control inhibit the ability to have an orgasm during intercourse, although they usually can ejaculate through masturbation or other stimulation. Their worries are often unconscious, and they need professional help to resolve them. Therapists usually use conversation to help people understand their worries. They may also suggest exercises to help each partner relax and lessen attempts at control. In most situations, the issue is essentially the man's to sort out.

> **My husband has trouble with premature ejaculation. He's tried behavioral techniques for the problem and things have**

gotten better. But I've been wondering if there's any medication that will help.

Behavioral therapy is the traditional treatment for premature ejaculation. It involves teaching men to become more attuned to preorgasm sensations and to do exercises that help them maintain control (see box titled "Behavioral Therapy for Premature Ejaculation," below). Behavioral treatment produces significant improvement in about 90% of cases.

Currently, there is no medication specifically designed to treat premature ejaculation. Some doctors have speculated, however, that antidepressant drugs may help with the problem, given that delayed orgasm is a common side effect of some antidepressants. For example, a study published in 1993 in the *Journal of Sex and Marital Therapy* reported that when a group of male volunteers took 50 milligrams of the antidepressant clomipramine (Anafranil) 6 hours before intercourse, it did delay ejaculation. Several men I have treated who did not do well with the behavioral exercises found this drug to be very helpful. The new group of antidepressants (Prozac, Zoloft, Paxil, and Effexor) also delay orgasms in many men and women; however, these medications need to be taken continuously to be effective. Although the practice of using a drug because of the benefits of its side effects is questionable, often people who have suffered with premature ejaculation for years may have a symptom or symptoms of depression as well. For such individuals, a short trial of medication might be conducted to see whether it is helpful. I should emphasize that many men have had the most dramatic results with one of the new antidepressants (e.g., Prozac, Zoloft). These men may not have been depressed, but they dreaded any sexual contact because of the worry about premature ejaculation. Their enthusiastic relief is compelling, and I feel that it is important to let people know that this is an option, and to discuss the pros and cons. I have seen men who recognize that there may be some unknown side effects from the drugs, but who say that the change in their self-esteem in feeling sexually competent is worth the risk to them. Similarly, I have talked with men who felt that they did not want to have a "pill" change their sexuality, but rather wanted to try and learn better control through the behavioral approach.

Behavioral Therapy for Premature Ejaculation

Premature ejaculation—coming too fast or too soon, or having no control—affects about 25% of men. Most suffer in silence, convinced that they are unique in being so affected and dreading the consequences of self-exposure. Dozens of complicated explanations for premature ejaculation have been offered: if a man comes too fast, it means that he is withholding, that he doesn't like to give, that he has deep-seated problems, and/or that he needs long-term therapy.

Forget all of these theories. Men who come too quickly need *coaching* and *training*. They need guidance to help them learn better control, and reassurance that all of the awful things they have felt about themselves are exaggerated and have become a reinforcing hindrance. I have treated many patients who suffered from premature ejaculation—men in their late teens and 20s who feel terribly embarrassed about their lack of control and who shy away from close relationships because of the shame they feel. I've also seen couples who have been driven to distraction with worry—the woman convinced that it must be her fault, that she is unattractive or that her husband or boyfriend really does not love her. Even couples who are committed and loving may find that sex gradually becomes filled with dread and disappointment and that self-esteem is slowly eroded by a growing conviction of personal failure.

Here are the facts about premature ejaculation:

* Orgasm is a reflex; control (like control of bladder and bowel) can be learned.

* For many men, there are no psychological causes, although the worry and shame lead to enormous distress and difficulties.

* There is no physical abnormality that results in coming too quickly.

* The idea that the man is selfish and is only focusing on his own satisfaction ignores the feelings of failure and the diminished pleasure that result from having premature ejaculation.

* The more a man worries about coming too quickly, the worse the problem becomes.

* Thinking about a baseball game (or some other distraction) does not work—and neither, for that matter, does the anesthetic jelly that is sometimes advertised.

Treatment Plan

The idea behind treatment for premature ejaculation is to help a man learn to stick with ever-increasing amounts of arousal. This principle runs counter to what many men believe is the problem ("I just get too aroused too quickly"). With guidance, a man can learn what it takes to control his orgasms.

The following plan is effective for most men within 4 to 6 weeks. The "exercises" can be done alone or with a partner. Often, I see men who have avoided relationships because of embarrassment about coming too rapidly and who want to gain more control in order to feel more confident. For many men who are already in a relationship, solo training is preferred initially because it makes them feel under less pressure. Finally, some couples welcome undertaking the project together.

First phase. Frequency is absolutely key. Doing these "workouts" at least three times a week is part of their success. More is better!

* Masturbate until you feel you might come.
* Stop and wait 60 seconds (use the second hand of a watch).
* Start again and time how long it takes until you feel you might come.
* Stop and wait 60 seconds.
* Repeat this four or five times; the last time, let your pleasure build and allow yourself to come.

Focus all your attention on the pleasurable sensation in your penis, and learn your own body signals that tell you how close you are to coming. Practice this for 2 to 3 weeks.

Second phase. You'll notice that it will take longer to get to the point of coming. This lets you know that things are changing.

* Masturbate until you feel that you are close to the "inevitability point" and then slow the stimulation so that you keep yourself at the same level. Here the task is to keep yourself at a constantly high level of arousal. You may have to slow your stroke considerably and at times even stop—but try to keep the arousal at that very high point. *You will suddenly realize that after a period of time, your threshold for coming will rise, and you will be able to stay with the heightened feelings.* Your goal is to keep this going for 20 minutes.
* Get to know your PC *(pubococcygeal)* muscle! This is the muscle you use to stop your urine flow midstream. Learn what it takes to contract it voluntarily, and practice—a

lot. You can then experiment to see what happens if you contract this muscle, or contract and then relax it, during your high excitement. Men vary in their responses. Some find that the contraction aids in control, whereas others find that alternating contraction and relaxation makes the difference. Still others say that learning to contract the PC muscle gently and progressively gives them the control.

* Once you feel consistent control, you can move to intercourse. Try the same approach: initially not much moving with your penis in your partner's vagina—a lot like the techniques you practiced with your hand. You'll have to concentrate on keeping the focus you learned, and you should expect that the initial few times may feel like you have lost the control you achieved.

Premature ejaculation is common but fixable. The key is to stick with the training I've outlined here in a consistent, frequent way. The exercises are not hard to take—certainly they are much easier than the hours of aerobics so many people do religiously. The battering to a man's self-esteem when he feels that he can't count on his penis is awful. Premature ejaculation no longer needs to be suffered alone—it can readily be treated.

I've been dating a man who is a widower, and I hope one day that we will get married. We have one big problem, though: He's impotent. When I first found out, I attributed it to a million different causes—nervousness, shyness, lack of practice. I even suspected he might feel as if he were being disloyal to the woman he had loved and lived with for so many years. But this has been going on for a year now. What's the prognosis for our romantic life?

This sounds like a problem I recently confronted in my practice. A former patient phoned me and explained that she'd become involved with a man whose wife recently died. She liked him a lot but was frustrated because he was unable to get an erection. I suggested that they come in for counseling together.

During our initial meeting, they related how they'd met at an adult education workshop. It wasn't long before they were seeing a great deal of each other. However, she noticed that he was shy about expressing affection and didn't make sexual advances. One night she asked him to stay over at her apartment. Although they tried to have intercourse, he was impotent.

When I asked Michael (not his real name) to tell me about that evening, he said he had no idea what the problem was. He felt embarrassed and ashamed. I then asked about his wife and her illness. He told me that they'd been happily married for 12 years when she developed cancer. At first, her doctors were able to control the disease through chemotherapy. Then it spread with a vengeance. His wife became more and more incapacitated, and during a 3-year period she suffered painfully before dying.

Michael hadn't really spoken to anyone in detail about this experience. During our one-on-one session, he became distraught as he described their relationship. He talked about how devastating it was to see the disease take over his wife's body and spirit. He felt helpless and overwhelmed by her physical pain. For the last 2 months of her life, he was at the hospital with her constantly, but there was nothing he could do to save her.

Because he'd held his feelings in for so long, Michael was emotionally exhausted. He'd been so busy for so long taking care of his wife's needs that he'd neglected his own. By talking and bringing his feelings to the surface, Michael was eventually able to accept his wife's death.

The following week, his friend called me and asked, "What did you do?" It turned out that since that session, Michael had no difficulty getting an erection. He wanted to have sex every night, and she said she was overwhelmed. "Is it okay to say, 'No'?" she asked me.

The lesson here is how easily many situations can be improved relatively quickly. Therapists and patients often believed people with sexual dysfunction need long-term therapy. However, if your friend had a healthy sexual relationship with his wife, effective short-term therapy probably would be enough to alleviate the problem. Not everyone experiences a rapid cure, but the chances of starting a satisfying physical relationship are good.

If your partner was impotent during his marriage before his wife became ill, however, there may be a medical problem or he may need to probe more deeply into the feelings that are blocking his sexual impulses.

> **I'm 33, happily married, and have two children. A few months ago, I totaled my husband's car. Shortly thereafter, he began to have difficulty getting an erection. He won't talk about it, but I think he might be angry with me, and that is causing his impotence. Is this possible?**

I'm afraid so! What happens between partners on a daily basis can have a powerful effect on sexual responsiveness. When anger is not expressed directly, it can come out indirectly in symptoms such as headaches, ulcers, and, yes, impotence and the inability to climax.

Talking about this with him may help. But from what you say, I think a third party is needed to help create a safe climate to discuss what has happened. The direct approach is what I would aim for first: "I really feel bad about wrecking your car—but I feel even worse about the fact that our sex life seems to have been so affected. I really miss the physical closeness with you and I don't know what to do. Would you consider seeing a professional with me to see if we can make things better? I would really like that."

While the words obviously have to fit with your style, what I am suggesting is communication that is not accusatory, blaming, or judgmental. If you can keep the expression of your position clear, it's more likely that your husband will be able to respond. Remember also that the first try may be a bust; people often feel very defensive and cannot hear what their spouse is really asking. Let a little time go by and then try raising the topic again.

> **How common is impotence? Is there ever an underlying physical cause?**

Impotence affects about 10% of men, and physical factors are often involved. A careful evaluation must include consideration of both physical and emotional contributors. Impotence can be a source of considerable pain and suffering, causing shame, low self-esteem, and anxiety. Its effect is so powerful that sometimes even a single incident can lead to a reinforcing cycle of failure. When a man is unable to have an erection, his partner often feels confused and worried that she is somehow the cause. Social situations in which sexual jokes are told become excruciating. Although the man may not talk much with his partner about the issue, it is invariably on his mind almost all the time, which only makes the situation worse.

Possible medical and physical causes of impotence include diabetes, thyroid disorders, neurological damage, side effects from medications, and malfunctions of the pelvic blood vessels (see "Impotence" section in Chapter 8, pages 113–115). That's why it is so important to have a thorough urological evaluation if impotence develops. Choose a physician who is familiar with the current methods of assessment. The evaluation should include the following:

* Evaluation of blood pressure and blood flow in the penis
* Blood tests to assess testosterone levels
* Evaluation of nerve function in the penis
* Nocturnal penile tumescence test, which detects the occurrence of erections during sleep

If a physical problem is found, a variety of treatment options exist; see the box titled "Treatment for Physical Problems With Erection" at the end of this chapter.

I have had diabetes for many years and have now become impotent as a result of the complications of the disease. I've tried everything, but nothing seems to help. I'm really worried that my marriage is going to fall apart.

Erectile problems in men (and orgasm difficulties in women) affect about 20% of people who have diabetes. It is an illness that affects many different systems in the body. Small blood vessels become damaged, and changes may occur in nerves that transmit sensation. It is these last two effects that can create sexual problems. To maintain an erection, three systems have to be working in sync: production of the hormone testosterone, blood vessels that are flexible and open, and nerves that transmit the electrical messages from the penis to the brain. Often with diabetes, there may be a mixed picture: erections may occur but be less reliable, and then the associated worry about whether the erection will last leads to a cycle of anxiety about performance. What starts off as a physical problem is compounded by the emotional reactions to it. The frustration and embarrassment of not being able to get an erection are often overwhelming.

You say you've tried everything—I assume that means you've had counseling that focused on behavioral techniques to address your sexual functioning. It also is essential that you be seen by a urologist who can evaluate for physical causes.

Treatment for Physical Problems With Erection

Nonsurgical Options

If physical problems are found, a recommendation may be made for *intrapenile injection* of medication—a technique that reliably produces a good erection that lasts about 30 minutes. Although men often shudder at the thought of doing this, they get used to the shots quickly and are thrilled not to have to worry about performance. In fact, in some men in whom no physical problem has been detected but in whom anxiety is prominent, intrapenile injections may be used as a "backup." Simply knowing that there is something that can produce a reliable erection often relieves the individual enough so that erections occur on their own.

Another treatment option is the *vacuum device*, a plastic cylinder with a pump that creates a vacuum. This is placed over the penis, which fills with blood "passively," and an elastic band is then slipped off the cylinder onto the penis to create a workable erection. Although somewhat cumbersome, this device can be an effective nonsurgical approach.

Penile Implant

A *penile implant* is a mechanical device that is surgically placed in the shaft of the penis. There are several different types, but the most commonly used has a small pump located in the scrotum that allows the implant to be inflated when needed. When an erection is desired, the man simply squeezes on the scrotum and the penis becomes erect. The penis increases in length and diameter. When the erection is no longer desired, the implant is deflated and the penis returns to its flaccid state. Be assured, it's quite effective and not at all as strange as it sounds. Sometimes sensation is lessened, but most men report they don't notice any changes and that orgasms are pleasurable.

Although the idea of an implant is sometimes disturbing to both men and women, there is no reason that having an implant should interfere with your sexual relationship. If you have a caring partner, you both will be happy with the renewed sexual contact. Approximately 90% of men with implants report being satisfied. At this point, 25,000 are inserted each year.

Before having this procedure, you need to know as much as possible about it, because there are some disadvantages. First, the procedure is not reversible. The implant can be removed, but a natural erection will never again be possible. Also, if the pump fails, you have to have another one put in. Finally, some men can never accept the notion of something "foreign" inside their penis.

If you are seriously considering an implant, ask your urologist to refer you to two or three couples who have experience with the device and talk with them about what it is like. Ask about how it works, how it looks and feels, and whether there were any surprises.

Note: Although I have stated that implants may help impotence caused by diabetes, there are times when the disease itself makes this impossible. The blood supply may be so bad that the surgery may not be feasible. There may be problems with healing, and infections and tissue damage in the penis after healing may make it necessary to remove the implant. Careful discussion with the physician is *extremely* important.

Chapter 4

General Sexual Functioning

*D*espite the depiction in the media that everyone is "doing it" and has no worries about sex, I continue to be reminded by the questions I am asked just how much ignorance still abounds when it comes to people's bodies, sexual anatomy, ideas about what is "normal," and the conviction that these insecurities have never been expressed by anyone else. Information can be a source of comfort and reassurance, especially when it comes to ideas about how rapidly one should get aroused, whether size matters, how to "make" your partner come, feeling responsible when your partner does not come, and wondering whether it is okay to bring up a fantasy.

Information about how the body works gives many people an understanding that is helpful. The questions that follow relate to how the body works sexually. These topics are covered:

* Positions for intercourse
* Intensity of orgasm
* Faking orgasms
* Simultaneous orgasm
* Postorgasm "collapse"

* Trouble having orgasm
* Lack of excitement
* Inability to have a second erection
* Nipple erection
* G-spot
* Pain in the penis
* Pain with intercourse
* Allergy to semen
* Oral sex and yeast infection
* Too much vaginal lubrication
* Sex during a period
* Lubrication and the pill
* Smoking and sex
* "Too much" sex?
* Air trapped in vagina during intercourse
* Penis size

What is the best position for a man and woman to reach orgasm?

There is no one "best" position to achieve climax: It varies from woman to woman, man to man, experience to experience. There are many components involved in sexual stimulation and enjoyment. First, to have an orgasm, it's essential that you be comfortable during sex.

Anatomy plays a major role in what position you prefer. The greatest concentration of nerves in women is in the clitoris, and any position that provides clitoral stimulation will enhance orgasm. The labia (vaginal lips) are sensitive to stimulation, as is the opening to the vagina. Most men find the head of the penis to be the most sensitive part, although the entire shaft responds to stimulation.

Changing positions will vary the angle of your pelvises to create direct clitoral contact or let the head of the penis rub directly against the vaginal wall. Many women enjoy digital stimulation of the clitoris during intercourse. This is easy to do if the man enters from behind and reaches around to touch the clitoris with his hand.

But, as I said, this may not be best for all women.

Whatever position you choose, focus on the physical sensations of lovemaking and try to let your body move in response to the feelings. Relaxation is a very important part of letting go; try to be aware of your individual needs to promote this.

Guide to Sexual Positions

While exploring new positions can be fun and can open up new experiences, some of the acrobatics should be reserved for those who are skilled gymnasts. Most people have a few favorite positions, and learning which work best for you is a matter of being open to experimenting. Listed below are some sources you may find useful.

Books

* *Sexual Happiness: A Practical Approach* (Yaffe and Fenwick 1988)
* *The Ultimate Sex Book* (Hooper 1992)
* *The Illustrated Manual of Sex Therapy, 2nd Edition* (Kaplan 1987)

Videos

* *Sexual Positions—Beyond the Missionary Position* (Polonsky and Dunn; FOCUS INTERNATIONAL)

Is it possible to increase the intensity of one's orgasm? Mine don't seem to be anything like my wife's.

There is no scale by which orgasms are measured; people are different, and they respond in different ways to sexual stimuli. If you feel dissatisfied with your level of arousal, there may be aspects of your sexual relationship that you can enhance to add to your enjoyment. Consider the following questions:

* Do you know what raises your level of sexual arousal?
* Are you able to tell your wife what you would like her to do?
* Do the two of you spend enough time attending to each other's physical needs?
* Do you feel comfortable masturbating? If you do, have you noticed what actions or stimuli can affect your orgasm?

If you answer no to any of these questions, think about exploring these issues with your wife. What I try to underscore is that sexual satisfaction requires more than a mechanical meeting of two sets of genitals; it involves learning more about your own responses and then sharing this information with your wife. It may be that you two need to communicate better during sex.

> **Can a man tell if a woman if faking orgasm? I need to know my new boyfriend better before I can feel relaxed enough to climax. In the meantime, I don't want him to feel inadequate, so I'm faking it.**

Physiologically, there are certain changes that occur in a woman's body during sexual arousal. The first visible change is vaginal lubrication, which is followed by a thickening and lengthening of the vagina. The clitoris also becomes enlarged, though at the height of sexual arousal, it retracts and appears to have become smaller. The nipples may also become erect.

As orgasm approaches, respiration and heart rate usually increase. Muscles may tense and the skin may feel more sensitive until climax takes place. This is accompanied by a series of rhythmic muscular contractions in the vagina and uterus. Involuntary sounds and facial expressions often occur simultaneously. The sensations vary in intensity, depending on the individual and the situation.

Mechanics aside, any woman who is determined to fake it and has a little acting ability can do it. Although I don't recommend it, faking orgasm is common. Your question makes me recall a scene from the movie *When Harry Met Sally*, when Meg Ryan demonstrated in a restaurant how to fake an orgasm, and someone at a nearby table called out, "I'll have what she's having!"

The second part of your question is very important; the burden of feeling responsible, inadequate, or abnormal is a heavy load to carry. This is where talking really helps. If your concern is that he feels inadequate, you might say just that! Tell him, "I'm worried that you feel you're not doing your job if I don't come. Really, it's not up to you. I need to know you better before I can feel comfortable letting go." I know this sounds trite, but when people are able to put their concerns into words, it usually results in their feeling better. If your boyfriend were the one asking this question, I would encourage him to ask: "You seem to be having a good time when we make love, but I worry that you don't have an orgasm. Is there anything I could do differently?"

My boyfriend and I are in our late 20s. We want to get married, but we're concerned because we have not been able to achieve simultaneous orgasm. What can we do?

First off, I hope that other considerations are involved in your decision of whether to get married. As for your question, the belief that simultaneous orgasm is a requirement of a good sexual relationship is an idea whose time has long passed. I would encourage you and your boyfriend to stop focusing on performance and "perfection" and switch your orientation to having fun. While simultaneous orgasm can be gratifying, it is by no means a necessary accomplishment. For many couples, this time is one of discovery, learning what each likes and enjoys and finding ways to share this knowledge.

As soon as I have a climax, I feel drained and completely collapse. Is this normal?

People vary greatly in their individual responses to sexual arousal and climax. The feeling of extreme relaxation that you experience is one of the very pleasurable parts of being sexual. In Victorian literature, when someone would have an orgasm the word to describe it was "spent." Many individuals seek the release that accompanies sexual arousal and climax.

> **I don't always have an orgasm during sex, although my boyfriend occasionally brings me to orgasm afterward. Why can't I come like other women?**

You *are* like other women. Clinicians report that around 40% of women don't reach orgasm during intercourse. I wonder if the two of you have silently agreed that something is wrong with you, rather than recognizing what feels special and exciting and using your imagination to broaden your range of activities.

Many couples learn a variety of approaches to provide satisfaction for the female partner, which may include shallow intercourse or the man caressing the woman's genitals with his fingers or stimulating her clitoris with his lips and tongue. Some women report reaching orgasm from stimulation to their nipples, as well. All these behaviors are "normal" and may be used separately or together to increase your arousal.

You might also take some direct control by stimulating your clitoris yourself while you are having intercourse. Try positions that make this possible. It is really limiting when couples believe that it is one person's responsibility to elicit all responses. Rubbing your clitoris while having your boyfriend's penis in your vagina can feel great—a real joint effort!

The fact that you *do* reach orgasm indicates that physiologically everything works. The two of you may find with time and experimentation that you can have an orgasm during intercourse, or you may be one of the large numbers of women for whom intercourse does not provide enough stimulation.

Medical causes of orgasm difficulties may include the following:

✳ Men and women with diabetes may have difficulties having an orgasm.

＊ Medications may inhibit orgasm. (If you were orgasmic and then stopped after being given a particular drug, the drug may be causing the problem. Check with your doctor.)

During intercourse I don't get very excited. Is it possible I have too much tissue between my vagina and clitoris?

The answer is no. It sounds as if there are other factors that keep you from getting aroused. There is no way to pinpoint a cause, and many factors can be involved, including the following:

＊ Lack of information about your body
＊ Fear that sexual feelings are not okay
＊ Worry about losing control

There are many factors involved in discovering sexual feelings. Some are related to attitudes and values in one's family; others are related to self-image and self-esteem (feeling good about oneself and one's body). Encounters and experiences that are part of growing up may facilitate or impede sexual expression. I would suggest reading some of the books listed in the appendix ("Information Resources") at the back of this book. These are self-help books that contain much useful information and suggestions for getting more in touch with your sexual self. If you are interested in trying to master this yourself, make sure that you set aside regular time to practice the techniques. If it does not help, I suggest you seek professional counseling—making sure that the individual has expertise relating to sexual difficulties.

My lover and I would like to have intercourse more than once, but he says he can't have a second erection. Is there anything we can do?

Let me explain the refractory period in men. Unlike women, some of whom can have several orgasms in rapid succession, once a man has an orgasm, he is usually unable to have a second erection and orgasm for a certain period of time. This can vary from a few minutes to many hours; teens usually have a refractory period of minutes, but it increases with age. There is a great deal of individual variability, and often a new relationship provides an emotional excitement that seems to override some of the delay.

Having addressed the mechanics, let me raise a few other questions. Do you feel that your boyfriend has sufficient control over his orgasm? If he has early ejaculation, you both may wish to have intercourse again because you felt that it was over too soon (see the box "Premature Ejaculation" in Chapter 3). How about the time you both spend before starting to have intercourse? Do you focus on sensual and sexual touching that can keep you both at high levels of sexual arousal for a longer period? Do you take turns stimulating each other, thereby prolonging your sexual experience?

Many couples regrettably are too focused on moving to the genitals, stimulating them, and having intercourse. In the process, lovemaking is over quite soon. By learning more about each other's sexual feelings, you may invent new ways to provide each other with pleasure before, during, and after intercourse.

Is there a way to stop my nipples from sticking out? It's embarrassing to be examined by a doctor, and worrying about it makes them stick out more.

What you describe is a normal reflex and I doubt that you can control it. The nipples, like the penis and clitoris, contain erectile tissue, which under certain circumstances becomes engorged with blood. You might try deep, slow breathing as a way of relaxing.

I've read that every woman has a specific part of her vagina called the G-spot, which must be stimulated to have an orgasm. Is this really true? Where exactly is this G-spot?

About 40 years ago, a gynecologist named Ernst Graefenberg thought that he had identified a place in the vagina that is highly sensitive and produces very intense sexual arousal. This "magic" place, known as the G-spot in his honor, is said to be a tiny collection of blood vessels and nerve endings no larger than a dime, located along the upper wall of the vagina. Ever since Graefenberg's announcement, researchers have been studying and debating whether there is a G-spot. Books have been devoted to the subject and videos produced attempting to demonstrate the phenomenon, including female ejaculation. In a study reported in 1986 in the *Journal of Sex and Marital Therapy*, researchers found that for a small percentage of women, there is an area of special sensitivity in the vagina. For the majority, however, they found no evidence of the G-spot.

Intense sexual arousal and enjoyment usually is centered in the clitoris—and the brain. The biggest turn-on comes from being with someone you like and wish to please, and who feels similarly about you. Figuring out what "buttons to push" is more suited to programming a VCR. Sadly, too many people are influenced by sensational reports that a certain technique will "drive your woman wild" or "make her scream with ecstasy." While I encourage mutual exploration and discovery, I urge people to remember that sex is not the Super Bowl.

> **When we make love, my husband complains he experiences some pain in his penis. Although afterward he says it is nothing, I know he is worried. He refuses to see a doctor because he is embarrassed. What could be causing this?**

Without knowing more about the nature and exact location of the pain, I can only offer some possibilities.

Pain on the surface of the penis may be caused by a skin condition—an ingrown hair, a small pimple, or an inflammation of the foreskin (if your husband is uncircumcised). These minor infections are easily treated, usually with antibiotics.

Pain in the urethra (the opening in the penis that connects to the bladder) could signal an inflammation. Most likely, your husband would also feel a burning sensation when he urinates. The cause could be an infection of either the bladder or the prostate. In this case, he would need an exam and test for bacteria and appropriate antibiotic therapy.

Pain during erection is a condition known as Peyronie's disease. In these cases there is a hardening of some of the tissue in the penis that bends the penis and causes pain. If this is the case, your husband should consult a urologist.

Pain during orgasm usually signals an infection of the prostate. Again, he should see a doctor.

> **Lately I've been avoiding sex because it's become so painful. My husband and I always had a pretty good sex life, but the last few times we had intercourse, I noticed a discomfort when my husband thrust deeply. What could this be?**

Pain during intercourse is not uncommon for women and may mean one of several things.

If you are not fully aroused, your vagina may not be lubricated and lengthened enough when the penis enters it. As a result, you would feel some irritation.

If you are aroused but still feel pain, you may have an inflammation or infection of the cervix. One possibility is pelvic inflammatory disease, a nonspecific diagnosis that describes an infection in any part of the reproductive tract. Usually the cause is a sexually transmitted infection, such as chlamydia or gonorrhea.

If the pain occurs only around the time of ovulation, you may have an ovarian cyst. These cysts are mostly benign, but sometimes they twist or rupture, causing severe pelvic pain. Fibroid tumors, also usually benign, may grow on the uterine wall and cause pain.

You may have an intestinal inflammation that is irritated by deep penile thrusting.

Finally, an ectopic pregnancy, in which a fertilized egg attaches to a fallopian tube instead of the uterine lining, could also be the culprit. Pain in this case, however, is constant and severe and requires immediate medical attention.

Your best bet is to see a gynecologist for a complete evaluation.

Whenever my boyfriend's semen comes in contact with my skin, I break out in a rash. It goes away in a few hours, but I'm worried about what it is doing to the inside of my body. It's gotten to where my anxiety is hurting our sex life. What can I do?

First, try having him use a condom so that no semen touches your skin. Because the rash goes away quickly, it probably is harmless. In terms of what is happening inside your body, do you notice any itching or pain in your vagina? There is sometimes a chemical incompatibility between a man's semen and his partner's vaginal secretions. This can lead to fertility problems but has no other significant consequences.

Semen is not toxic, and you don't have to worry that you are being harmed. This is an inconvenience and nothing more. I suggest keeping a towel nearby and wiping the semen off your skin as soon as you can. Or go to the drugstore and buy prepackaged cleansing cloths formulated for the genital and anal areas. You may also try a little aloe skin lotion.

Every time I perform oral sex on my wife, she develops a yeast infection. Her doctor suggested that it is probably caused by bacteria on my tongue. Is there a medication that might help?

It's possible that oral sex changes the acidity of your wife's vagina. She should try using a white vinegar douche after sex, using one tablespoon of vinegar in a douche bag with water.

I produce too much vaginal lubrication during sex. It is clear and odorless, but there is so much of it that it lessens my sensations. My doctor says I have no yeast or bacterial infection. I lubricate so much that at times I have to have a towel under me during sex.

When it comes to vaginal lubrication, there is a wide range of variability—just as with everything else. Some women feel they produce too little. You have landed on the opposite end of the spectrum.

You might try placing a tampon in your vagina before lovemaking begins. It will absorb much of the fluid, and can easily be removed before intercourse.

> **I find that I often feel very aroused during my period, but I don't know if it's okay to have sex at that time. My husband is interested. Please could you give us some information?**

From a health point of view, intercourse during your period should cause no problems. Women often worry that their bleeding makes them unappealing. You already have reassurance from your partner that he's not put off. Other men sometimes find the sight of blood on their penis disturbing. It really comes down to personal preference.

An additional note: Menstruation can give a couple a sense of excitement and freedom because there is less risk of pregnancy (assuming that the woman's periods are regular). Remember, however, that intercourse during menstruation is not *completely* safe, as sperm have been known to remain viable inside the vagina for as long as 5 days. Thus, if intercourse occurred near the end of a woman's period, she could ovulate while the sperm were still viable.

> **Ever since I started taking the pill, my husband and I have noticed that I don't get as lubricated during sex. Is this possible? What should we do?**

The answer is yes. The pill certainly can cause dryness in the vagina. The contraceptive works by altering your hormonal balance with a mixture of the hormones estrogen and progesterone. That shift in body chemistry may result in physical changes for some women, including a lowered sexual interest.

You don't complain of not feeling aroused, so if a lack of lubrication is your only problem, there is no need to stop taking the pill.

You could use any one of a number of excellent commercial products, such as K-Y Jelly. Water-based lubricants are best.

You may also discuss your complaint with your gynecologist and consider using a different oral contraceptive or using a non-oral method. As with any medication, it is important to review with your physician the current position regarding long-term side effects and to consider going off the drug periodically for a few months.

> **Someone recently told me that smoking affects sexual performance. I never knew that. Is it true?**

Many people do not realize that smoking damages small blood vessels, and this obviously includes the blood vessels of the penis. At this point, there has been much documentation of the effects of smoking on the cardiovascular system. When this happens, erectile difficulties can result. One wonders if a label on cigarette packaging saying "Warning: The Surgeon General Has Determined That Cigarette Smoking Is Harmful to Your Erection" would be effective as a deterrent.

> **Is it possible to "burn out" your body from too much sex? My wife and I are healthy, in our 30s, and make love almost every night.**

Consider yourselves lucky and enjoy! There is no danger of "sexual burnout." Studies have shown that the more regularly and frequently people engage in sex, the more likely they will be sexually active well into their 80s. It's a myth that sex is depleting; there is no scientific basis for this claim. In fact, people often say that regular sexual activity makes them feel better and more energetic.

> **This is a little embarrassing to ask. When my husband and I are having sex, and he pulls out his penis, it sounds as if I am passing gas. What is it, and how do I stop it?**

During the thrusting of intercourse, air sometimes gets trapped in the vagina, and the noise you hear is the air being released. There is nothing bad or wrong with this and, of course, there is nothing you can do except forget about it.

> **My husband is very self-conscious about the size of his penis. I've told him that I am sexually satisfied by him, but he wants to try to have it surgically enlarged. Is there such a procedure, and are there harmful complications?**

It is sad how many men are plagued with this concern, and it seems as if nothing will reassure them. I know of no reliable method to enlarge a penis. Some of the devices I have read about—such as a vacuum that pumps up the penis to a larger size—theoretically may work. But they have not been tested rigorously, and I suspect they could damage the penile blood vessels. Distending the penile veins would result in loss of ability to hold erections.

Some plastic surgeons will graft fatty tissue into the penis to widen it. Patients interviewed on television about the changes all reported increased self-esteem. It sounds too risky to me, however. I'd never do it because my worry about surgical complications would outweigh any appearance concerns. I have spoken to many men whose adolescence was torture because of their belief that their penis was too small. The sensations of pleasure that one can derive from one's penis are totally unrelated to size, however. The problem is that these men become obsessed with their supposed inadequacy and have great difficulty focusing their attention instead on the feelings that are produced when their partner touches their penis.

The myths about penis size have been around in a variety of forms forever. I remember seeing the "forbidden" drawings in Pompeii depicting a man with his penis on one side of a scale and gold on the other. The guide told us that this was what it meant to be "worth its weight in gold!" Pornographic movies and pictures only add to the concern, because all the models are selected precisely for their abnormally large penises.

Bernie Zilbergeld has dealt with this topic in a wonderfully humorous way. Here's an excerpt from his book *The New Male Sexuality:*

> Penises in fantasyland come in only three sizes: large, extra large, and so big you can't get them through the door. "Massive," "huge," and "enormous" are commonly mentioned in fiction. Not only are penises huge to begin with, they can get still bigger during intercourse. "She wailed in hot flooding ecstasy. It went on and on, one climax after another, and as Craig's penis lengthened unbelievably, his semen erupting within her, she wailed again, this time in unison with him." With that penis expanding the way it was, it's no wonder everyone was wailing. These organs that might be mistaken for phone poles are not mere flesh and blood but "hard as steel," "hard as a rock," or a "diamond cutter." Something that could cut a diamond, the toughest substance in the world, must really be hard. One wonders whether we're talking about making war or making love with these tools. There is, of course, no joy in a penis that's sort of hard, semihard, or "only 70%" erect. (p. 50)

In his book *Ask Me Anything*, Marty Klein says that a penis should be "small enough to fit through a door and large enough to be found in the dark" (p. 17). I know that, as with many beliefs about one's body, the individual suffers with his or her perception, regardless of any outside reassurance. It's a source of considerable pain for many.

Chapter 5

Fears

"**A**m I normal?" and "Is this okay?" seem to be universal concerns. In the sexual arena, worry about such things is intensified when people don't express these concerns. Because people often have such a deep-seated belief that something may be wrong with their bodies, they are often reluctant to seek out information from an informed professional—which might change their view of themselves. It is as if they have decided that their inner reality is unchangeable, with the conviction that a doctor would only confirm their opinion of themselves. I am constantly impressed by how these secret concerns cause a huge amount of pain and are not shared with spouses or friends.

Topics covered in this chapter include the following:

* Self-consciousness about body
* Too-large labia
* "Dirty" talk
* Sex without a relationship
* Masturbation in front of girlfriend
* Sex and drinking
* Husband wants wife to have an affair
* Husband needs to have penis touched to get erect
* Marriage and masturbation

* Sexual dreams about other women
* Suddenly he can't keep his hands off me
* Uncomfortable sex after menopause
* Woman always has to make the first move
* Man is affectionate with his male friends
* Husband thinks he's bisexual
* Ex-boyfriend had genital warts

> **I am terribly self-conscious about my body. When I look at myself in the mirror I find fault with just about everything. I worry that my husband does not find me attractive, and I can't bear to make love with any lights on. I feel so weird but I can't stop these worries.**

Almost all people have something about themselves that makes them cringe a little—such as a narrow chin, thick ankles, coarse hair. Many people are able to develop a balanced view and recognize attributes that offset perceived limitations. Many people suffer from low self-esteem and are plagued by perceived imperfections in their bodies. This problem affects both men and women, although I suspect that women are more verbal in expressing these doubts. I have seen many people in my practice who are very attractive by any standards and yet feel that they are basically ugly and unappealing. It is of little use to try to persuade them that they are mistaken. It is often necessary to look at childhood family experiences to understand the roots of this problem and lessen its effects.

I believe that the primary source of a sense of well-being is the reciprocal interaction of parents and children; the child is excited about some accomplishment, and the parent reflects and validates the feeling. The reverse holds true where parents may not "mirror" children's good feelings, and those children grow up with an impaired view of themselves. Often one or both parents have been critical, unsupportive, or devaluing in powerful ways. Kids are unable to protect themselves against these attacks on self-esteem, and they incorporate their parents' negative opinions into how they view themselves.

Letting your husband know how awful you feel may be a source of some comfort, but I suspect that you need counseling to truly break this pattern. If your body-flaw obsession has you avoiding social situations because you're embarrassed to be seen, it's time to seek professional help. A good therapist will help you understand the roots of your negative feelings and help you free yourself from a considerable burden.

> I recently became sexually active and I fear I have a bizarre problem. My labia are too big. They seemed to get in the way during sex. I feel like a freak. Is there anything that can be done?

Just as some people have big ears or noses, so genitals vary in shape, size, and color. There is nothing wrong with your labia. I encourage you to talk with your partner about your feelings and recognize that this is who you are. It might be helpful to talk to your gynecologist and discuss your concerns. I know that there have been articles describing plastic surgery to reduce the size of the labia, but I would be very cautious about considering that kind of surgery.

One of the problems is that most women rarely, if ever, get a close look at other women's genitalia. By comparison, men often have the experience of showering together or of changing in locker rooms where there are opportunities to see what other penises look like. Many of the sexual handbooks available have pictures and illustrations you could consult to get some idea of the range of variability in this area (see the appendix ("Information Resources") at the end of this book).

> My boyfriend likes to "talk dirty" when we are making love, but it makes me feel very uneasy. What's worse, he wants me to do it, too. The idea makes me feel silly, and I think it's bizarre. Do you think I'm too uptight?

My only rule when it comes to sex is, "Usually, if it feels right, it is right—for you. If it feels wrong, don't do it!" If you are uncomfortable doing something with your boyfriend, whether it is using explicit language, trying a new position, or having sex when you are not in the mood, be true to yourself and decline. Relationships require give and take, with both partners showing respect for each other. Going along with something that simply isn't right for you is not likely to leave you feeling good about yourself or the relationship. You certainly won't enjoy sex if you feel that you've been forced into something. Finally, ask him why this turns him on.

> I'm 24 years old, single, and attractive. I wonder whether I have a problem, because I find that I seek out men simply for a sexual relationship. And after we have slept together a few times, I don't want to see them anymore and am driven to find someone new.

Many people are terrified by the idea of becoming committed or "dependent" on another human being. They turn off any relationship that shows even a remote possibility that it could endure. While I can't know the specific causes of your fear-avoidance pattern, for many there may be family patterns in which strong emotional ties were associated with pain and loss. Here are two specific reasons why the behavior you describe may occur:

1. Being desired sexually by someone else may temporarily let you feel that you are worthwhile, liked, admired, and valued. However, you may fear being unworthy of those compliments, and this may provoke you to end the relationship and begin the process anew with another partner.
2. You may associate having sex with closeness and acceptance—being loved by another human being. In this case, the sex may not feel very good or satisfying, but just having another person interested in you and attracted to you creates an illusion of being valued and important. That feeling of well-being is not lasting, however. As doubts creep in, your sexual interest may shift to another person.

It is very hard to figure this kind of thing out on your own—I would suggest talking to a counselor.

> **My girlfriend wants me to masturbate in front of her. I'm not sure I really want to. Do other people do this?**

The simple answer is yes, some people do masturbate in front of one another. But for all those who do, there are just as many people who don't, either because they're uncomfortable with it or because it doesn't happen to appeal to them.

It's better for you to tell your partner what's on your mind than to feel pressured into doing something with which you're not comfortable. Letting go in front of another individual requires confidence and trust; if you feel that, this may be an activity that brings you closer. Once you've explored your feelings, do it only if you feel ready, willing, and safe.

> **My boyfriend and I only have sex when he's been drinking. I know that alcohol makes a person's hormones rise, but does that mean he's not attracted to me the rest of the time?**

I'm not aware of any rise in hormones associated with alcohol. If anything, alcohol is a drug that usually leads to a dulling of sensations and a lessened ability to function. It sounds to me as if your boyfriend needs to drink to relax and feel less uptight about making love. I don't think it has anything to do with you.

It's important to realize that many men are quite nervous and afraid when having sex (contrary to the popular belief) and often worry about being adequate in their performance. I suggest that you ask him why he thinks he needs to drink. Having said that, I recognize that if he is nervous about his performance, it is also possible that he will not welcome talking about it. People often feel that asking them about why they do things is a criticism of that activity. An opener might be, "Look, there is something I would like to talk about. I have felt confused that each time we make love, it seems that you need to drink. When you do that, something changes about your personality that is a little uncomfortable for me. What do you notice the drinking does for you?" You might add that you know that alcohol is supposed to relax people, and if that is the purpose, try to find a way that the two of you could relax without using alcohol. You might suggest something like a body massage, where the focus is on something that feels pleasurable and relaxing rather than becoming "sexual" immediately, with all the attendant pressure about performance.

> **After 15 years of marriage, my husband is badgering me to have an affair. At first I was amused. But then I realized he was not just fantasizing about this. He really wants me to sleep with someone else. Can you venture a guess as to why?**

Without knowing more about your husband and your relationship, it is very difficult to understand what is going on here. I have learned that relationships evolve continually, that there is an ebb and flow of intensity, and that changes occur when one or the other partner is strongly affected by either an external change in life or a powerful internal struggle. Sex may become a stage on which many complicated feelings get played out. I don't know whether your husband has been feeling less interested sexually and feels bad about that or whether he is concerned about changes in his life and having thoughts about having an affair himself. He may feel conflicted about these thoughts and is encouraging you to do what he is thinking. That way, he does not have to feel bad about his unexpressed wishes.

I suspect that it is more complicated and should be addressed professionally. Clearly you are not comfortable with the idea, and it seems out of context with how your relationship has been over time. I suggest telling your husband that it feels strange to you and that rather than exciting you, it makes you feel uncomfortable. If talking together does not lead to some opening up on the topic with increased understanding, I would encourage you to see a counselor jointly to help clarify what this may be about. I would suggest putting it in a positive light—which is that your relationship is too important to expose to a risk that you barely comprehend.

> **My husband used to get an erection just by looking at me. But after 25 years, he needs manual stimulation to make his penis erect. Is this a signal that he is not attracted to me anymore?**

Don't take it personally. Many older men require their penis to be touched directly to become aroused. People are often struck by this change and disturbed by it. Men often notice that when they were younger, the mere thought of a sexual encounter would cause a strong erection. When this does not happen, unfortunately many men come to the conclusion that there's something wrong with their penis, and many women conclude that their partners are no longer attracted to them. This is where caressing and touching can be extremely important. You may be thinking, "He never needed to do *that* before." Couples too often focus on getting their genitals to work together and forget that the realm of sexual pleasure is wide. They forget to explore the varieties of touch, to see the skin as a vast, sensuous organ.

The fact that it takes your husband longer to develop an erection or to have an orgasm could add to your sexual enjoyment; you have the opportunity to savor a more prolonged sexual time together.

> **One evening when my husband was away on a business trip, I masturbated and enjoyed it. Now that he's back, I still do it, though we have sex several times a week. Do you think there could be something wrong with me?**

Despite our new "enlightenment," discomfort and misinformation regarding masturbation persist. At least people no longer think that they will go blind, but the question about its normality persists. Masturbation offers people an opportunity to derive considerable enjoyment and pleasure from their own bodies. Often, people are confused because orgasm with masturbation may be more intense than with a partner. This really is not surprising. It is your body: You know it best and therefore know what to do to create the most intense feelings. However, the popular belief is that once you're married or involved in a significant relationship, masturbation should cease.

We know that between 40% and 50% of individuals continue to masturbate throughout life. In fact, many people who are having an active, enjoyable sexual relationship are more likely to masturbate than those who are not. The only time masturbation could be a problem is if it is replacing sex with a partner. However, from your description, it sounds as though you and your husband have a healthy sexual relationship. I wouldn't worry about it. Feeling comfortable with your body and giving yourself sexual pleasure will enhance your experiences with your husband.

> **I've been happily married to a wonderful woman for the past 8 years. Lately, though, I've been having sexual dreams about other women. I feel confused and guilty. Does it mean that I'm falling out of love with my wife?**

It's completely natural to have dreams—even explicitly sexual ones—about someone other than your partner. In fact, it's quite common. During a night's sleep we go through several periods of REM (rapid eye movement) sleep, during which time we become sexually aroused. The REM stage of sleep is also when we dream, which is why our nightly thoughts are often of a sexual nature.

Many people also enjoy fantasizing or daydreaming about sex with different people. For some, this can stir intense guilt, and they work hard to suppress such thoughts. What they don't realize is that sexual dreams and daydreams are effective ways of expressing sexual urges. Dreams are a function of your uninhibited thoughts and are special in that they are not bound by the usual rules of logic and social decorum. Rather than feeling guilty about them, you might think more about their content during the day and see if they reflect desires that you have been unable to express to your partner. Some couples enjoy sharing each other's dreams. The important point is not to take the content too literally. Sometimes a dream may involve anger at a partner, while your feelings may in reality have something to do with a conflict at work or with someone else. In the dream, expressing these feelings toward someone familiar feels safer.

> My husband and I have been married for 10 years. He's 42. For the first 2 years of our marriage, we had sex practically every night, but after the kids were born, we cut back. Now for some reason, his pattern has changed, and we have sex much more frequently. He can't seem to keep his hands off me. I'm not complaining, but I wonder if this is normal for a man his age.

If the change in your husband is sudden and appears to be out of character, have him consult his internist and ask for an endocrine workup. I don't want to alarm you, but out-of-the-blue, distinct fluctuations in sexual behavior sometimes are associated with a pituitary tumor. An unexplained spike in a person's sexual drive also may indicate a psychiatric illness or brain disorder or could be a side effect of some medications.

Although you should rule out all other possibilities, the most likely explanation for your husband's behavior is what used to be called a "mid-life crisis." Although many of these catch phrases have been so overused that they have lost much meaning, the phenomenon relates to that distinct awareness that seeps through one's consciousness and says, "I have a finite amount of time left, and that scares me!" I recall someone telling me that you know you've hit mid-life when you start counting down. The realization that there is limited time left in our lives is uniquely disturbing when it hits. I have been struck while perusing birthday card racks by the ever-increasing number of cards for the 40-something crowd that focus on the infirmities of getting old.

One way people may reassure themselves that they will not be taken over by the aging process is to jump into a frenzied bout of sexual activity or have a sudden desire to change careers, buy a new car, take up an unusual physical activity such as skydiving, or return to earlier passions.

There may be other psychological explanations. Have there been any significant changes in your husband's life? Are certain stresses less of a problem than before? The answer to your question would best come from your husband. Why not ask him what he thinks is going on?

> Two years ago, my father died. Last year, my mom began dating. She just called me, quite upset. Apparently, she and a man she has been seeing attempted intercourse recently, but she experienced a lot of pain. Her doctor told her to "just relax." She was offended, but doesn't know where else to turn.

Your mother might be experiencing changes that occur with menopause (the cessation of regular menstrual periods). Natural declines in the production of estrogen can make the vagina less elastic and the skin thinner and decrease vaginal lubrication. Many, but certainly not all, women also find it harder to get aroused. The capacity for orgasm is unchanged, however.

ERT (estrogen replacement therapy) reverses some of the changes caused by menopause, but ERT isn't for everyone, and your mother should discuss its pros and cons with her doctor. Her doctor could prescribe a topical vaginal estrogen cream that may make a difference as she moves into a more active sexual relationship.

There has been much controversy about ERT. Some believe that it may increase the risks of breast and ovarian cancer. Others feel that the benefits in terms of protecting the heart and slowing bone thinning outweigh those risks. It helps to get information from more than one source and to then try to make an informed decision.

Additionally, if a woman has not had intercourse for 6 months or more, she may experience a narrowing of the opening to the vagina. This could be the cause of your mother's pain when attempting intercourse. The next time, she and her partner should move things along slowly and use a lubricant such as K-Y Jelly.

It's also true that many individuals who enter into a new sexual relationship later in life find that they experience the same kind of uncertainty, worry, and anxiety that they had when they first became sexually active. This is often disconcerting and confusing. They may ask themselves, "What gives? I've been sexually active for decades." Developing a sexual relationship later in life, however, can be every bit as anxiety-producing as it was in one's late teens or early 20s. Concerns about being accepted and worries about competence are normal. Some older people may even find it confusing to have sexual desires, because as a society we have pretended for so long that the older we get, the less interest we have in sex.

That is yet another myth that's perpetuated without questioning. Masters and Johnson and other scientists have clearly shown that healthy individuals maintain sexual function well into their 70s and 80s. Yes, there are physical changes that require some adaptation. But individuals who enjoyed sex in the earlier parts of their lives will likely continue to enjoy it as they grow older.

> **I really have a problem! Increasingly, I am the one who has to initiate sex. When we first got married, my husband was the spontaneous one. But now after 4 years, if I don't make the first move, nothing happens. I worry that he is not attracted to me, or worse yet, that he is having an affair. What do you suggest?**

Your fears are not at all unusual and are probably groundless. My bet is that you've fallen victim to the sexual myth that men are always ready and eager for sex and that if your husband is not initiating sex with you, he must be actively seeking it elsewhere. In truth, it is normal for an adult's sexual drive to vary enormously, depending on life's circumstances. How a person responds, performs, and enjoys sex is influenced by how busy, preoccupied, or tired he or she is.

Sexual disinterest, however, is not something you should ignore. One thing that can help is to look for misconceptions, false notions, or myths about sex that you or your husband may have unconsciously picked up that may contribute to his apparent lessening of desire. Here are some factors to consider:

1. *He may feel under pressure to always have great sex.* Men and women today often worry themselves sick about their sexual performance. They believe they are expected to know what pleases their partner and to be totally concerned about their partner's satisfaction and enjoyment. Many feel they must constantly offer their partner erotic excitement and novelty, and that pressure often makes them feel like retreating and hiding instead. Check out titles of magazine articles in popular magazines—"Are you married to a good guy who is sexually boring?" Take a look at how sex is portrayed in the movies: people with perfect bodies and not a moment's hesitation or uncertainty, who always know what their partner desires.

   You may have to reassure your husband that sex doesn't have to be great all the time. Being open to different scenarios and intensities is more realistic. After all, even a "quickie" before falling asleep can offer enough closeness and comfort to temporarily fulfill each other's need for emotional and physical closeness.

2. *Outside pressures may be dampening his libido.* Because sex can often relieve tension, logically you'd expect that the more stressed out you are, the greater your desire for sex should be. That's not how it works. Pressures of all kinds—work, school, child rearing, health, money—influence a person's sexual drive, often profoundly and usually adversely. Even worse, when a man or woman is worried about work, he or she may shut down emotionally instead of letting the partner know what's going on. Sadly, we can't selectively turn off our emotional responses, so sexual feelings dim, too.

3. *He may have clinical depression.* Depression is a medical illness that affects one's mood or spirit. The most common symptoms are changes in sleep pattern, level of energy, appetite, mood or self-esteem, and a decreased sexual drive. Without proper medical treatment, which can include talking to a

therapist and taking medications, the severity of the symptoms may increase. He may expect you to solve his problems and be disappointed that you can't or may secretly blame himself for not being "good enough" for you.

Being in a close relationship may also be associated with unanticipated changes. Once people marry, they become more like "family" to each other, and they begin to react to comments more defensively, as if they were uttered by a critical or nagging parent rather than a loving and caring spouse. When this happens, sexual interest may wane. Who, after all, wants to get close with a nagging complainer? Most often, the spouse has no awareness that he or she is being perceived this way, and unless the couple talk openly about the way they view each other, they are stuck in the dark.

As you can see, there are several possibilities. So what should you do? First, talk with your husband, but choose your approach carefully. Don't whine or accuse. I would *not* suggest saying something like, "I was talking to Susan the other day, and she and Don make love four times a week. So, what's wrong with you?"

Instead, try to describe what you are feeling and to exchange information—not barbs. You might say, "There is something I want to talk about. It is hard for me to discuss, and I worry that you might get hurt or angry. I love you very much, and I am confused and sad about the changes in our sexual relationship. It seems to me that you are less interested in sex and that I often have to initiate it. I worry that you don't find me attractive anymore. What do you think?"

Inhibited Sexual Desire

In cases of inhibited sexual desire, everything works but interest is just not there. This problem affects between 20% and 30% of couples at one time or another.

Possible Causes

* Depression
* Medication
* Marital difficulties
* Childhood sexual abuse
* Illness, either short- or long-term

What to Do

* Professional help is usually needed
* Antidepressants may help
* A combination approach is often useful: individual/couples/sexual therapy

I have noticed that my partner is very affectionate with his male friends. He hugs them a lot, puts his hands on their shoulders, and, it seems, has more physical contact with them than other men have with their friends. I've heard of married men who are gay. Should I worry?

These are tough times for men. Women often claim they want a "sensitive" man, but if he's *too* sensitive, he causes a stir. We have much to learn about the emotional needs of men and how to foster vulnerability and strength in them. Little boys are allowed to be sensitive until they reach the age of seven or eight, at which point society begins to send blatant signals that it isn't acceptable.

For too long, men have been discouraged from displays of affection and emotion. I think it's refreshing to find a man who can show his feelings. That ability is probably part of what attracted you to your partner in the first place. My hunch is that he's expressing feelings of affirmation and closeness with his male friends—and nothing more. Unless you have other reasons for thinking your husband may be gay, appreciate this warm, gentle side of him.

> **My husband thinks that he is bisexual. He feels attracted to men but has not acted on this. I am trying to be open-minded but feel freaked out. What is going on?**

Of course you're upset, and you probably feel totally confused. Recognize, though, that it took guts for your husband to tell you, and I believe that reflects basic trust in your relationship.

Many people have feelings and interests that are bisexual (feeling a curiosity about and attraction to the same sex). For most, it remains a private fantasy or daydream. Here is a brief overview of bisexuality:

* Many people have a sexual curiosity and interest in same-sex activities as well as heterosexual activities, and this may have no implications for the primary relationship.
* In some cases a man may have had homosexual feelings for a long time but suppressed them or was too frightened to act on them. A man in these circumstances may marry, hoping that the feelings will disappear, only to find that they don't.
* Some couples engage in bisexuality as another avenue of adventure. (This is called *swinging*.)
* Masters and Johnson describe a phenomenon they call *ambisexual*, which refers to people who have either heterosexual or homosexual relationships without any strong preference.

This is a particularly difficult topic to handle on your own, and a third party would probably diffuse the intensity and add some clarity to what is going on. When confronted with this problem, I suggest a joint meeting to hear how the couple has struggled with the concerns, then schedule an individual meeting with each partner in an attempt to understand the meaning of the attraction. Usually, getting things out in the open is a huge first step—very difficult to do, but enormously relieving. From that point, I try to build on the strengths of the relationship to help a couple work this out.

My ex-boyfriend had warts on his penis. I don't see any on myself, but could I have caught them from him? I've heard cervical cancer is caused by these warts. Is this true?

Genital warts are an STD caused by human papilloma virus (HPV). The virus makes an infected cell divide at an increased rate, causing a wart to form. These warts are common and are highly contagious. The problem is that they may or may not be noticeable. In men, they can be found in the urethra (the passage from the bladder to the penis) or on the shaft of the penis, the scrotum, or the anal-genital area. In women, they can be found on the labia, anal-genital area, vagina, or cervix.

The virus has been implicated in cervical cancer. Women who have sex with a man who has had more than six sexual partners have a greater risk of having abnormal cervical cells, probably because of the increased risk of exposure to this virus.

Genital warts need to be taken seriously and treated by a physician familiar with current treatments. (See a board-certified dermatologist, urologist, or gynecologist.) Treatment may involve medication to destroy the warts or freezing or burning the warts off. It is essential that infected individuals be examined annually by a physician to check for recurrences. Women with genital warts should be particularly vigilant about having a diagnostic Pap smear test at least once a year.

Sexual intercourse should be avoided until treatment of the warts is completed. Condoms and spermicide offer only limited protection. This is a serious condition. Do not let embarrassment stop you from seeking appropriate medical care.

Chapter 6

Relationships and Values

A close, open relationship based on trust and a capacity for having fun both in bed and out is the key to exciting, fulfilling sex for most people. Sex is complicated, though, and may be affected by either subtle shifts in the relationship or changes in the emotional state of yourself or your partner. Problems arise when we do not, or cannot, express ourselves clearly to our partners.

Figuring out your partner's needs and wishes is often difficult, though essential if a relationship is to feel reciprocal and sustaining. *Intimacy* became a buzzword in the 1960s and has now lost much of its original meaning. In my view, being close with someone involves being able to feel accepted, valued, and safe; it means feeling known and understood and being able to convey a similar understanding to your partner. This is not a fixed, immovable state, and there are constant shifts in a relationship. However, when there is a basis for the openness I have described, it is always possible to return to that openness and feel that your partner is a valued and trusted part of your life. When there is a feeling of trust and safety, you are more likely to be able to take charge and talk honestly with your partner. If you make that a priority, there's a good chance that you won't miss out on the happiness and well-being you deserve.

71

Whether we like to admit it or not, we all run our lives with an internal set of guidelines or values. We begin to have a sense of what we like or don't like, what sorts of things are important and have value, what we are comfortable with, and what we wish to avoid or reject. Our original families are the primary source of our expectations. It is here that we view adults and how adults behave, and it is in this context that we learn what to expect from others, what makes us feel good in a relationship with other people, and what causes us pain.

Adolescence is a time to begin defining ourselves. We challenge parental rules and values, push limits, and try to figure out what we will incorporate for our own values. This process continues in early adulthood, when we physically move away from parents and family and begin to make choices for the paths we will follow. Developing sexual relationships is an important part of this growth; initially, people are propelled by intense hormonal shifts that result in strong sexual feelings. Eventually, the complexity of being in a committed relationship begins to exert more of an impact, and the need to define who we are, what we like and dislike, and who makes us feel good or bad becomes more central.

In this regard, people are surprised that when they were younger they experienced an openness and desire to experiment in all aspects of relationships, and as they get older they have a greater need for stability. Throughout life, there is an ongoing process of getting to know who you are and defining the values that work for you. Sexual values are only one component.

The questions presented in this chapter are related to values, attitudes, and differences in preferences:

* Humans and lifelong partners
* Son is gay
* Sexual chemistry
* Boyfriend says partner doesn't initiate sex enough
* Boyfriend has uncontrollable erections
* Husband won't make eye contact during intercourse
* Diminished enjoyment of sex

* Husband reads pornography
* Wife has poor self-esteem
* Husband is having an affair
* Couple doesn't have sex
* Wife wants to know about husband's sex with ex-wife
* Wife dreads sleeping with husband
* Wife wants more variety
* Wife doesn't remember what husband likes
* Partner is turned off by oral sex
* Headed for divorce, but sex is great
* Husband wants sex even if wife isn't in the mood
* Inability to have sex in parents' home
* Husband's "liberation" exhausts wife
* Husband and his friends talk about other women in front of wife
* Wife has started a business and husband can't get an erection

Please settle a debate a friend and I are having. She says human beings are programmed to have more than one lifelong partner and that's why so many people cheat. Is this true?

Your friend's reasoning is too simple and frankly not even accurate. In a survey by researchers at the University of Chicago, released in 1994, the most surprising fact was the degree to which couples were monogamous and the higher level of sexual satisfaction among these couples. New sexual relationships are enormously exciting to many people. But to suggest that we are "programmed" to have serial lovers is absurd. (Of 3,432 people interviewed, fully 75% of men and 85% of women said they were faithful.)

Monogamy as an institution endures because the companionship and security it offers create an intimacy that cannot be found elsewhere. Your friend may find it easy to rationalize having an affair by saying that it is "natural" to want more partners. Frankly, in my experience, people who have many affairs are the ones who complain most about feeling empty and depressed. As time goes on, it gets harder and harder to find the thrilling, intense excitement they seek in each new lover. They yearn instead for what they are missing: the fulfillment and personal joy that are possible in an enduring relationship.

> I have a son who is 42 years old, has been married for 18 years, and has three children. The other day he told me that he and his wife were getting divorced. I asked him if there was another woman. You can imagine my shock when he replied that it was in fact another man! I don't approve of homosexuality, but he is my son and I love him. What should my attitude be?

Shock sounds like an understatement! You are going to need time to digest this new information, but while you do, try to remember that he is the same person as he was before you knew about his homosexuality, and more than ever, he needs you to be supportive and helpful.

It sounds as if your son has chosen to do something courageous. I have no doubt that he struggled to control his homosexual feelings for a long time, until finally he realized that he could not make them go away. That is why, despite the consequences for himself, his wife, and his children, he has declared his feelings openly.

It is impossible to predict how his announcement will affect his children. Certainly, each member of the family should be offered professional help for dealing with this new information and the enormous changes that it will bring. Remember, though, your son's homosexuality should have nothing to do with his capacity to be a good parent. If he was a caring, involved father before this revelation, he will be after it.

> What is it about "chemistry" in sexual relationships? I've noticed that sometimes sex feels good with a guy, but the relationship goes nowhere, and other times I am with a guy I like and who cares for me, but sex is a dud. Why?

Sexual chemistry is complicated, variable, and elusive and cannot be explained in a neat formula. Certainly, many men and women find sex can be great only in the context of a committed relationship. For others, the opposite is true: Sexual excitement and pleasure are heightened when there is no commitment and they know little about their partners' inner lives. In such cases, learning too much about a lover makes sexual interest wane.

Sexual chemistry also varies in importance from one person to another. Some men and women won't even consider becoming lovers unless there is an "animal attraction" right from the beginning. Others must spend a lot of time with someone before they can develop a sexual bond. Then there are people who are willing to try sex with someone they are not attracted to physically, because of an attractive personality. Often to their surprise, they fall in love and this becomes the engine that then drives their sexual feelings. There's truth to that old saying that the brain is the most important sexual organ!

Relationships often involve compromises; if you are with someone about whom you do not feel excited sexually, you have to ask yourself if the other qualities make up for what you feel is missing. I have seen many people who have had many very exciting sexual partners before marriage who believe that, although sex with their spouse is somewhat uninspired, commitment, reliability, and character more than make up for the lack of excitement in their sex lives. It is a personal choice, and it is probably different in various life stages.

> My boyfriend says that I don't initiate sex enough. I don't feel ashamed or guilty about sex, but he is right in his observation. I enjoy sex if he starts something. Is there anything I should do?

I would encourage a respect of your differences without defining your level of interest as problematic. It seems as if the two of you have a satisfying sex life; you both participate and get pleasure from it.

There could be many reasons to explain your hesitancy to initiate sex. As I have repeatedly stressed, there is no perfect relationship, and as you have mentioned, you do respond to your boyfriend and you like what you're doing. It might be helpful to get a consultation with a trained therapist to help you both see if there are any obvious things you might be missing.

In his 1988 book *Sex Is Not Simple*, psychiatrist Stephen Levine talked about the ways people "borrow" sexual comfort from a confident partner and experience discomfort from an apprehensive one. Relationships in their most positive form are reciprocal; your boyfriend may have the qualities that help you get in touch with your sexual feelings, while you may bring qualities that add something special to his life.

> I am dating a young man whom I like a lot except for one problem. He cannot control his erections. Whatever we do—shopping, walking, dancing—it is so obvious. He says he can't help it, it just happens. Sadly, I may terminate our relationship because of this.

People are frequently aroused during their daily activities. Most people simply enjoy the sensations and aren't bothered by them. Your boyfriend's involuntary erections make no statement about you or his feelings for you. If you think the erection is too visible, ask him to use underwear that has more support, or to wear loose-fitting, pleated pants. What you should be focusing on is how the two of you get along.

> When my husband and I make love, he refuses to make eye contact with me. He insists on positions so we can't look at one another, and he won't consider changing. I really like eye contact during sex, and I'm frustrated and confused by his attitude. What do you think is going on?

Sex means so many different things to people. But I hope I have conveyed my belief that sex can provide a way for two people to feel close and safe and have exciting sexual feelings. For that to happen, partners have to trust one another and be willing to engage in a give-and-take relationship.

Many people, however, find self-exposure uncomfortable. This may be an issue with your husband. Very often, the patterns of sexual behavior may mirror the "out of the bedroom" part of the relationship. I don't know whether your husband is unresponsive and insistent on his way in other areas, but if he is, the problem may be more relational and less sexual. It seems to me that you have a few options: You can put up with it; tell him you feel there would be more satisfaction for both of you if you participate more in lovemaking; or seek counseling. Frankly, I think counseling might be the best option, since it would offer you enough support to make a stand for what you need from the relationship.

> I seem to enjoy sex less than I used to. I don't know why. I love my wife very much and think she is absolutely stunning! I just can't seem to get excited about making love. I changed jobs last year and took on more hours. Could that be part of it?

Sounds reasonable to me! Time is scarce for many couples, resulting in people being overworked and "undersexed." So many couples are working harder than ever that I'm hearing more and more of the same complaint—either one or both partners are having trouble putting work aside.

There is no easy solution. Simply saying you have to make more time for each other does little good. However, I have a few suggestions that might help make you closer both emotionally and sexually.

Talk to your partner about how you can't seem to let go of job concerns and how you've noticed that the two of you are spending less enjoyable time together. Venting your frustrations may help her understand the depth of your problems and pressures. Getting her perspective may surprise you.

Consider trying to set up weekly "dates" where the two of you go to dinner (even pizza or sandwiches at the nearest diner). Try taking walks together or some activity that you have enjoyed doing together. It may sound corny, but sometimes scheduling this time makes a difference.

Is it possible to spend some time away with each other? This doesn't have to be something elaborate—sometimes one night at a nearby hotel where you can go to sleep early and spend some unpressured time together the following morning makes a big difference. To help get some time alone, some couples trade child care with other families, taking turns watching the children.

Try to set aside 10 minutes each day to talk about each other's day. Too often, people slide into an isolated state and forget the resources they have in each other.

I don't mean to oversimplify life's pressures, but some of these suggestions may help break the cycle of poor communication and bad sex.

> **During our 20-year marriage my husband has read several pornographic magazines each month. He keeps them hidden from me, but when I find them and confront him, he throws them away. It's only a matter of time, though, before he buys more. Those magazines make me feel inadequate, even though I think he has a problem.**

There are many different reasons men (and women) buy these magazines. Some of them are problematic and others are really harmless. Pornography *is* a problem for people who use it as a substitute for the usual give-and-take in relationships with a partner. Also, pornographic magazines and films that portray sadomasochism, bondage, and domination reflect, in my view, aberrant behavior. They are invariably demeaning to women and portray relationships in a power-oriented and debased way.

For some people, however, the magazines simply satisfy a curiosity, a wish to look and see. Some men and women have a hard time allowing themselves to entertain sexual fantasies, and the magazines provide the permission and the freedom to let their imaginations go.

If your relationship is solid—and if your husband falls into the category of simply curious—my suggestion is that he keep the magazines discreetly hidden and that you not worry about them. Sometimes couples need areas of "privacy," and this may be one of them.

> My wife's self-esteem is lousy, and I'm sure that it's a result of her mother's constant criticism. The situation has gotten so bad that it's beginning to intrude on our sex life. I tell my wife that she is beautiful and that I love to touch her. But she doesn't believe I mean it. What can I do?

You're probably right when you say that her mother's criticism is the source of the problem. The power of parental disapproval can be very strong. When someone has grown up with parents who were very critical, it's hard for that person to imagine that others don't think of her just as negatively. It's what I term the "my mind is made up; don't confuse me with facts" syndrome. Your wife doesn't believe you when you say you love her, because she isn't able to right now. She has instinctively re-created what was so painful about her childhood in her relationship with you. The roots of these feelings go way back, and they're not going to go away on their own.

> After 12 years of marriage, I recently discovered that my husband is having an affair. Our marriage has been pretty good, with the usual ups and downs, and we have two children. I am devastated. I feel angry, hurt, betrayed, and confused. Is it possible to repair our relationship?

The emotional shock of discovering a spouse's affair is staggering. Everything feels as if it has been turned on its head. Besides the stress in coping with this betrayal, you have to continue to be there for your kids, providing for their needs when you probably least feel able to do it.

In my experience, sex usually isn't the motivating factor for an affair. There are often other problems in a relationship that provoked the spouse to stray. Here are a few suggestions for what to do now:

1. You both need to see a professional to help you uncover the real reasons for your husband's affair. During a crisis like this, it is unlikely that either of you can be objective. My experience with many couples in this situation is that the hurt and anger on their own make productive discussion impossible and often result in escalating fights with recriminations and damaging attacks.

2. Your husband has to stop the relationship with the other woman, at least while the two of you try to figure out what it means, why it happened, and what you feel about your relationship. I think it would be impossible to unravel your feelings for each other if he continues to be involved with someone else.

3. Throughout all this, you both need help figuring out how to provide a stable home for your children. This includes trying to keep usual routines and discussing the affair only in private. Acknowledge to the children that you are dealing with a difficult problem and that both of you are under pressure. They need to know that they aren't the source of the tension. Too many details are unnecessary, however, and at all costs do not try to get them to take sides.

Although the experience is one of the most devastating a person can go through, I have been able to help several couples understand what one or both felt was missing in their relationship, figure out ways that each could be more responsive, and go on to build on their strengths. This obviously is not always possible, and in those cases where it is not, I have tried to help people separate and deal with their sorrow, rather than split in anger and "demonize" the other person. I always try to keep in mind that there was usually a time when each had very different, positive feelings for the other, and to lose that completely is to abandon what was once good.

> I'm 30 and my husband is 47. We've been married for a year
> and we have a sweet marriage, but our sex life is horrible!
> Before we got married we made love often. Now we have
> sex less than once a month. If I don't approach him, forget
> it. He's told me that he's afraid he might not be able to get
> an erection. What can I do to improve our love life?

First, it's important to realize that you are not alone. Couples often notice a change in their level of sexual activity once they get married, and this often confuses them.

I have noticed that when people recognize they have made a commitment to each other, a strange thing happens: As they feel more like "family," they begin to interpret and react to their partners' actions and words as they would have reacted to incidents in their original family.

One issue to address, however, is your husband's concern about his performance. A man of 47 shouldn't have trouble getting an erection as long as he's in good health, is not taking medication, and doesn't smoke.

My guess is that, for some reason, he has developed performance anxiety. Men who experience this tend to avoid sex, letting more and more time elapse between making love. The more time that goes by, the worse his anxiety will become. Consider seeing a counselor together who can help you and your husband work through the problem. With guidance, you can both resume the fulfilling sex life you once enjoyed.

> I am remarried to a wonderful woman. There is only one
> problem. She asks many questions about my sex life with
> my ex-wife, which was super. I am afraid to tell the truth.
> Should I?

Some say that if your relationship is really good, there is nothing that a couple can't share. Frankly, I don't think that's true. A relationship is about sharing experiences, but there are situations in which "telling all" may stir up unnecessary hurts, insecurities, or worries. In your case I am not sure whether you are reluctant to talk about the fact that sex may have been more exciting with your ex-wife. However, without knowing more, I suggest that you listen to the inner voice that tells you *not* to talk about your former marriage. You might say something like, "I wish you would not keep asking about this. I would be more comfortable moving forward and focusing on the fact that we have our relationship now." Finally, do you understand why she wants to know?

> **I'm beginning to dread sleeping with my husband. I love him, but I just am not turned on by him anymore. Please help.**

Most couples find that their sexual energy, attraction, and interest vary dramatically over the course of their relationship. Passion seems always present when the relationship is new, frequent as the couple get to know each other, then more sporadic as they settle into a comfortable, committed relationship.

Typically, as the relationship becomes established, making love gets pushed lower and lower on the "to do" list, until concerns about things such as jobs, children, health, parents, and money crowd it out altogether.

Also, after being constant sexual companions for a while, couples can get stuck in the rut of thinking they know everything about what works and doesn't work for them. They let their sex lives get set into a pattern of routine: foreplay and intercourse, without spontaneity. Making love soon becomes another part of the weekly routine, safe and familiar without joy and ecstasy. Eventually, it seems expendable.

Another more subtle but common problem that long-term couples encounter occurs when one partner begins to recognize characteristics in the spouse that are connected to his or her original family. While the conscious association may be positive ("Mike can put people at ease the way that Dad always could"), there may be less-recognized negative connections that become activated during intimacy.

For example, if the wife remembers her own mother as critical and unsupportive, there may be times when she feels her husband is coming across the same way, even though that may not be his intention. During sex, her husband may say or do something that she misperceives as being critical, in the same way her mother criticized her when she was a child. That unconscious connection decreases her enthusiasm for sexual contact, at least for the time being. Over time, this emotional chain reaction may shut down her libido.

On the more pragmatic side, there are many "personal irritants" that may interfere with sexual interest. Hygiene is a big one. Often I hear about how a spouse may not brush his or her teeth or take care of cleanliness in a routine way. For some couples this may not be important, but for many it is.

Weight gain may contribute to a partner being turned off. Often the sensitivity around this issue may make it difficult to bring up. I have suggested to couples that they can provide encouragement for each other in a weight-reduction or exercise program, making it an activity they can both be involved in.

The way to find out if there is something about you that bothers your spouse is to ask: "Is there anything about me, my body, or my habits that you find is a sexual turnoff?" I remember one man complaining bitterly that his wife was not interested in sex. When I asked her about it, she told me she had asked him for years not to smoke a cigar before coming to bed, which was a complete turnoff for her.

> We have been married for 7 years, and our sexual relationship is basically good. I still find my husband very attractive, but I long for more variety. We only make love in bed. I think that changing the venue would add something. What should I do?

Have you talked with your husband about some of your ideas? Varying the place and time that you make love most certainly would spice up sex. I suspect that you and your husband have what is a common problem: You both wish for something different but feel embarrassed or awkward about saying so. You might try being assertive and making direct suggestions to your husband. This will require you to put aside your censoring self and take a risk. It's to be hoped that talking about your desires will bring you and your husband closer. Not only will you be sharing something deeply personal, but he may in turn express his own secret thoughts about things he might like to try. There are some very simple activities that can add something new to a "mature" relationship:

* Setting time to make love during the day. Most couples tend to make love late at night, when they are both drained and tired. Passion really wilts fast then.
* Taking a bath or shower together. You may have done that routinely earlier in your relationship, and then as you settled into day-to-day activities it may have seemed inefficient as you rush to get going each day.
* Giving each other a massage. This can not only be relaxing but can also provide a pleasurable time that need not result in sex.

Overall, my sex life with my wife is okay, but there's plenty of room for improvement. Here's the problem: When I tell her what I would like, she is very cooperative for a bit, then seems to forget and fall back into being very mechanical. When I ask her what things she would like to try in bed, she invariably replies that she doesn't know.

This reminds me of a scene in the movie *Annie Hall,* in which a man and woman are both talking to their therapists. When the man is asked how often the couple makes love he says, "Hardly ever—three times a week." When the woman is asked the same question she replies, "All the time—three times a week."

The point is this: Each partner's perception of the same situation can be wildly different. Your complaint is common; each spouse thinks the other does not listen. I suggest you confront this directly in a conversation. You might say, "Look, I'd like to tell you what I think happens with us sexually, what I like, and what I think could be better. I hope you can try to do the same with me."

It may seem unromantic to ask, "Do you like this?" during lovemaking. But it is direct and to the point, and it may be easier than trying to bring up the topic later on. One couple I counseled discovered that reading a sex manual together led to an easy, open discussion about variety. They enjoyed it so much, they read it one chapter a week and then put the new information into action.

> **I really want oral sex, but my partner is not turned on by the idea. What can I do?**

The first thing would be to ask your partner what turns him or her off about oral sex. Many people think of genitals as dirty or smelly, and this belief will obviously affect someone's interest in engaging in this activity. Not knowing what to do or how to do it adds to reluctance. In several of the books listed in appendix ("Information Resources") at the back of this book, there are illustrations and suggestions for various techniques. If cleanliness is part of the concern, bathing together and washing each other's genitals could be a new and interesting activity. You may be able to encourage your partner to experiment and see if there are ways you can enjoy oral sex. Because the mouth and the genitals are richly supplied with nerves, the potential for this being very enjoyable is high.

> **My marriage of 13 years is headed for divorce. The strange thing, though, is that sex continues to be great. It remains the one area where we feel good and are responsive to each other. To be honest, I don't understand this.**

The usual pattern is that sex mirrors what is going on in the relationship: When it is good, sex is very, very good, and when it is bad, sex is horrid. There are couples, however, who can separate sex from the interpersonal part of their relationship and have a wonderful time in bed, even as they treat each other terribly in every other arena. To be honest, I don't understand how this happens.

I wonder if the situation you describe really is a signal that all is not lost. Sex might be a nonverbal way of declaring that you two are still involved and connected to each other. I would strongly recommend that you see a couples' counselor to help you be certain before you sever the relationship.

> When I'm not in the mood to have sex, and my husband is, he insists that we do it anyway. He says I'm wrong to deny him, and he gets angry if I seem upset about it. Who is right?

As far as I'm concerned, *no* means *no*. You shouldn't be forced to do anything that you don't want to do. If one partner isn't interested, the other must respect his or her wishes.

I suspect that your problem is not a sexual one; rather, there seems to be an absence of compromise in your relationship and your husband's inability to tolerate frustration.

In addition, if you never feel interested in sex, you may want to ask yourself if you have reservations about your relationship in general, which are surfacing in the bedroom.

> My wife and I frequently visit my parents, who live out-of-state. Whenever we stay in their home, I lose all interest in sex. Is this unusual?

I will try to explain why and how this happens so frequently. The ties and bonds between parents and children are very powerful. Although we may grow up, move away from home, make independent choices, and follow a lifestyle different from our parents, we continue to feel strong emotional connections to them.

The unspoken messages and values that we learn are extremely powerful and continue to exert their influence despite our moving away from home. For many, although there may have been a warm, loving atmosphere during childhood, sexuality was a taboo subject. Often, parents gave mixed, if not negative, messages about sex, and these get reawakened during visits to parents.

A well-known family therapist, Dr. Murray Bowen, writes

about how he spent years figuring out what made his family tick, and yet all the clarity and insight he developed would disappear the moment he set foot inside his parents' house. Old, unwelcome responses and behaviors would emerge, and his newfound understanding would be lost in a cloud of confusion. Things would not return to normal until he was on the plane back to his own home.

I suspect that the "child" part of your personality takes over when you arrive at your parents,' and the disapproval that may have been communicated to you (often nonverbally) takes over. Talking about it with your wife may be a relief, and if you are able to find some way of seeing humor in the transformation, the discomfort may be lessened. Realize that it does not mean that you are having serious problems, and try to accept that sex may not be comfortable during these visits.

> Joining a men's group has suddenly made my husband want to experiment and try all sorts of new and different sexual activities. I'm getting worn out by the pressure. I want a break from his intensity.

It sounds as if his self-discovery has left out one important component—you! Discovering untapped inner potential can be very exciting and rewarding, but it sounds as if your husband has mixed that up with self-indulgence. He wants you to gratify his newfound sexual adventurousness without taking into account its effect on you.

Somehow you are going to have to spell out your needs and your limits in a direct, nonconfrontational way. You might try saying something like, "I feel this. . . ." or "It's okay for you to want to do that, but I'm not comfortable doing anything that doesn't feel right to me." This is one of those instances where the "informational" mode, where you spell out as clearly as you can where you are coming from, is better suited to resolution than the "reactive" mode, where you attribute selfish intent and inadvertently start a fight.

My husband and his friends make remarks about other women in front of me. My husband says that it's just guy talk, and I shouldn't take it personally. But I do. It makes me feel as if I'm not enough for him. Am I overreacting?

Your husband's saying that the comments that upset you are merely "guy talk" is his way of excusing himself for the behavior and avoiding a discussion that might result in his having to stop it altogether. He should take your concerns more seriously. I wonder how he would feel if you and your friends talked about the latest "hunk" while he was around.

I wouldn't recommend confronting him as he is making the remarks, because both of you will have your defenses up, and the situation is likely to end in a nonproductive argument. Think through what you want him to know about your feelings and how you would like him to change his behavior. Then, pick a time where you are not likely to be disturbed to discuss your feelings. You might start off by saying, "Look, there is something you have been doing that has upset me, and I would like to let you know how I feel about it." What often helps is having the goal of letting your husband know what it feels like to be in your shoes. If he responds defensively, try to stick to your focus, which is to have him understand your experience.

You might also mention any behavior that you have refrained from simply because you know he does not like it. A relationship is a two-way street, and it's important to know that each of you is willing to do things for the other.

The kids are grown up and out of the house, so a few years ago, I started a business that has become very successful. I've noticed that the better the business is, the less my husband is interested in sex. What gives?

A change in the balance of the relationship can significantly alter a couple's sex life. He may feel competitive with you, and while this is quite common in close relationships, couples often have a hard time acknowledging it. Your success and strength may threaten him, especially if his own career is winding down, and he secretly may be worrying that he is becoming weaker as you are "coming into your own." Frequently, such thoughts can lead to depression, with lowered self-esteem and diminished interest in sex. You might initially talk with your husband about the changes you have observed and ask for his ideas about their causes. However, the issue is a sensitive one, and it may be a relief to have a third person help put into words the meaning of the changes in your lives. Sometimes a few sessions with a counselor or therapist are enough to help a couple unload and feel better. In cases of severe depression, the person may need antidepressant medication, and most people are highly responsive to this treatment.

Chapter 7

Getting Help

*T*he good news is that people have many options for help that only 10 years ago were not available. The constant barrage of material in the media has served to educate (although also intimidate) people sexually. Rather than suffering in silence and wondering whether unsatisfying sex and poor communication are inevitable, people should realize that there are several sources from which help is available.

This chapter deals with the following topics:

* Self-help
* Finding a therapist
* What happens in sex therapy
* Sensate focus exercises

Self-Help

I like to encourage people to explore their own strengths and resources and to see whether they are able to solve problems on their own. The way individuals learn varies enormously. Some like to educate themselves, try things out on their own, and experiment, while others like more direction and need the safety of a counseling format to take some of the risks that change requires. Early in my practice, I would hear couples say, "We've read all the books, tried the suggestions, and they don't work." Initially, I wondered what I would have to offer that would be different—and realized that for many, having a supportive and encouraging "teacher" provides a context in which change can take place. If a couple's communication pattern has been open and collaborative and the relationship is on a sound footing, trying some of the following suggestions may be enough. If they don't produce results, there is always the option of seeking outside help. (Details on the materials listed below are provided in the appendix ["Information Resources"] at the back of this book.)

Problem: Low desire or difficulty having orgasm

Try This:

* *Becoming Orgasmic* videotape (Heiman and LoPiccolo; FOCUS INTERNATIONAL)
* *Becoming Orgasmic* (Heiman and LoPiccolo 1988)
* *The New Our Bodies, Ourselves: A Book by and for Women* (Boston Women's Collective 1992)
* *Female Sexual Awareness: Achieving Sexual Fulfillment* (McCarthy and McCarthy 1989)
* *Sexual Happiness: A Practical Approach* (Yaffe and Fenwick 1988)

Problem: Vaginismus

Try This:

* It is important to consult with a gynecologist and confirm the diagnosis. For some women, the hymen may be particularly strong, and intercourse might be difficult and

painful. However, minor gynecological surgery will correct this. Vaginismus is always associated with difficult and painful intercourse.

* *Treating Vaginismus* videotape (LoPiccolo; FOCUS INTERNATIONAL). This tape has a direct approach and provides practical suggestions. The use of vaginal dilators is recommended; these can be obtained from F. E. Young and Company, 1350 Old Skokie Road, Highland Park, IL 60035.

Problem: Premature ejaculation

Try This:

* *You Can Last Longer* videotape (Polonsky and Dunn; FOCUS INTERNATIONAL). In this tape, Marianne Dunn, Ph.D., and I discuss premature ejaculation and provide suggestions to cure it. Two couples demonstrate the technique, and many have found this to be enough to solve the problem.
* *The New Male Sexuality* (Zilbergeld 1992). This book provides good coverage of the topic and has well-written suggestions for mastering control.
* *ESO* (Brauer, Brauer, and Rhodes 1989). Although the emphasis in the title ("Extended Sexual Orgasm") appears to be on Olympic training, the book has good suggestions in the section dealing with premature ejaculation.

Problem: Erectile difficulties

Try This:

* A urological evaluation can rule out possible physical causes of impotence (see page 34 in Chapter 3).

* *Treating Erectile Difficulties* videotape (LoPiccolo; FO-
  CUS INTERNATIONAL). For anyone who wants to know
  what happens in sexually focused therapy, this is a good
  source. A simulated couple, in which the husband has erectile difficulties, consult a therapist. The course of treatment unfolds on camera, beginning with the evaluation
  process. The therapist is shown directing the couple with
  specific homework assignments, and the couple is shown
  doing the exercises.
* *The New Male Sexuality* (Zilbergeld 1992). This excellent
  book covers many aspects of sexuality and male psychol-
  ogy. Particularly helpful is a series of suggested exercises
  and role-play activities for couples.
* *The Potent Male: Facts, Fiction, Future* (Goldstein and
  Rothstein 1990). This invaluable text contains current information about the mechanics of erection, the tests
  needed to determine what is not working, and the medical,
  surgical, psychological, and behavioral treatment options
  available.

While the self-help approach may work for many, it does not
always lead to solutions. I have often heard from people that "we've
read all the books and followed all the suggestions—and they didn't
help." In these situations, what is needed is the opportunity to talk
with someone who is trained to help with sexual problems. With
an objective "outsider," people are often able to reveal much more
of their thoughts, worries, and observations. Having a comfortable,
safe place in which a conversation can begin makes the process of
change easier.

How to Find a Sex Therapist or Marriage Counselor

Finding a professional who is trained and knowledgeable in this
area is often difficult, for several reasons. People are reluctant to

ask friends or co-workers, because in so doing they will reveal trouble in a very private and intimate part of their lives. In many regions of the country, there simply are not that many therapists who are trained in sex therapy or couples counseling. If you are comfortable doing so, ask your family doctor, internist, gynecologist, or minister or rabbi to make a recommendation. In addition, many large hospitals and medical schools are equipped to make referrals, and some even have sexual dysfunction clinics.

Another option is to contact a professional association. Here's a list of relevant ones:

American Association of Sex Educators, Counselors and Therapists
11 Dupont Circle, NW, Suite 220
Washington, DC 20036

American Association for Marriage and Family Therapy
1717 K Street, NW, Suite 407
Washington, DC 20006

American Psychiatric Association
1400 K Street, NW
Washington, DC 20005

American Psychological Association
750 First Street, NE
Washington, DC 20002

Society for Sex Therapy and Research (SSTAR)
Blanche Freund, Ph.D., Secretary
419 Poinciana Island Drive
North Miami Beach, FL 33160-4531

Local professional associations (check your telephone directories in the business section)

Investigate the Therapist's Credentials

There's a wide variation in the background and training of sex therapists. First and foremost, you want someone who is licensed, has a degree from an accredited university or college, and is affiliated with a recognized medical institution or professional organization.

In the United States, any mental health professional or physician can claim to be a sex therapist, whether or not he or she has taken courses in the field. That is why you should ask detailed questions about credentials. Also, check with your state health department to find out licensing requirements.

Discipline Training Requirements

I am often asked to explain the difference between psychiatrists, psychologists, social workers, and psychotherapists. The issue is not as simple as describing the different training requirements and experiences. Empathy is something I believe cannot be taught. Making connections with patients or clients is often intuitive, and although training helps refine this ability, the innate personal qualities of the individual are of crucial importance. The following list briefly defines the training required for each of these disciplines.

Psychiatry

* 4-year bachelor's degree
* 4-year medical school degree (M.D.)
* 3- or 4-year residency training in hospital setting
* Licensing requirements (board of medicine)
* Specialty board certification

Psychology

* 4-year bachelor's degree
* Postgraduate training at either master's or doctoral level

* Clinical programs involve training in clinical settings, which can be hospitals or outpatient clinics
* Licensing requirements (professional associations and state boards)

Social Work

* Associate's or bachelor's degree
* May involve postgraduate training at master's or doctoral level
* Clinical placements in hospital and outpatient settings
* Licensing requirements (state and association licensing)

Psychotherapy

* This is a gray, poorly defined, and poorly regulated area. In many states, anyone can call himself or herself a psychotherapist and hang out a shingle.

When calling for an appointment or at your initial meeting, ask the therapist following questions:

* Where and for how long did you train?
* Did that training include clinical experience?
* Are you licensed or certified?
* What did that process entail?
* What professional organization do you belong to?

Some therapists will be open and forthcoming about this information, while others will become defensive. Trust your judgment when it comes to entering into therapy—and remember that a second or third opinion is fine. Therapy is a complicated process, and the "fit" between therapist and client is absolutely crucial. It does not matter if someone has impressive degrees and a great reputation if you don't feel that the match works.

Discussing a Treatment Plan

Discuss your treatment plan before you begin. Have as frank a talk as you are able. You want to know what to expect from therapy before you begin. Here are some key points to discuss:

Have you treated many people for this concern or condition?   A "no" is not necessarily reason to seek another therapist. There have been many situations where I have had to improvise as I go along. However, I feel comfortable telling prospective patients the limits of my own experience.

Can you give some idea about outcome?   Obviously there has to be latitude here. I find that generally I can make some prediction about outcome, though I am always impressed by the times I have been wrong. There have been many couples I thought would never improve who made rapid gains and others whose treatment I thought would be brief and simple with whom the opposite occurred.

Can you share some of your ideas as to what my problem is?   I am always turned off when therapists take a "just trust me" approach. It is reasonable to ask a therapist to share with you some of his or her ideas as to what is going on. I tell patients that I view therapy as a collaboration where we are working together to solve a problem. I often share my hunches, not because I know the hunch is right but to test out an idea. I need patients' feedback as to whether they feel I am on the right track.

How many visits will be required?   Initially, I meet with couples weekly. This gives us some continuity and also intensity. However, after a while, it is sometimes possible to spread out sessions and have more "homework assignments." Some problems can be dealt with quickly, but if difficulties in the relationship or more complicated personal issues come up, the time frame will change.

How much will it cost?   Therapy is not cheap! Some of the cost may be covered by medical insurance, although this is diminishing, seemingly daily. The fee range depends on the discipline of the therapist and also on geographic location. The range is probably between $80 and $200 per visit.

Therapy of any kind is a dynamic process. Underlying problems or new issues often surface during treatment, which may require more sessions or a variation in the treatment plan. That's why it is important that you evaluate the tone as well as the content of what a prospective therapist says in response to your questions. Is he or she brushing off your concerns? getting defensive? or reassuringly explaining various options and approaches?

A word to the wise: Avoid anyone who claims that his or her method will unquestionably cure every problem.

Trust Your Instincts

This is often difficult. When you seek therapy, almost by definition you are feeling vulnerable and uncertain, and it is difficult to challenge someone who sounds authoritative and expert. However, although a therapist may be good and reputable, he or she may just not be right for you. If the chemistry is off, it can affect the whole course of treatment.

Here are some questions to consider:

* What is it like for you when you visit the office?
* Is the therapist on time, or do you have to sit in the waiting room long past your appointment time?
* Does the therapist seem accessible or remote?
* Is the therapist responsive to your fears and anxieties?

Remember, you need to try to be your own advocate. If therapy does not seem to be working, you always have the option to stop and get a second opinion. It is hard for some not to worry about being a "bad patient" or hurting a therapist's feelings. If you have established a relationship with the therapist, it may help you to discuss what is bothering you and why.

What Happens in Sex Therapy

You don't have to *do* anything in the therapist's office! People are often terrified that they will have to demonstrate their difficulties with the therapist watching. My goal is to create a setting where people can feel safe, can be helped to put their concerns into words, can be educated about sex, and can be encouraged to share with their partners their worries and insecurities. Sex therapy, whether for individuals or couples, is all about talking. Its aim is to offer support, hope, an understanding of the problem, and, most important, detailed instructions for overcoming issues such as premature ejaculation, arousal difficulties, orgasmic response, painful intercourse, inhibited sexual desire, and many others.

It is natural that people would feel uneasy about going for counseling. It is uncomfortable and embarrassing to be expected to reveal to a perfect stranger the most intimate details of one's life. When a spouse is reluctant, I encourage him or her to consider attending at least one meeting and to reserve judgment about the process until after that meeting has taken place.

The first thing a therapist usually does is let the patient know that he or she is not alone. Statistics confirm this:

*   Roughly 10% of men suffer erectile difficulties.
*   Roughly 25% of men experience early ejaculation.
*   Roughly 10% of women find intercourse uncomfortable.
*   Roughly 40% of women don't reach orgasm during intercourse.
*   Roughly 30% of couples have inhibited sexual desire.
*   Roughly 50% of couples experience a serious sexual problem at least once.

The main therapeutic method is to shift the couple's focus away from *performance* and toward *pleasure and enjoyment*. The therapist is there to help the couple do that for themselves. How? By breaking sexual activities down to their smallest units—I call these "imaginary building blocks"—and then having the couple put the pieces back together. During the initial therapy, it's not uncommon for the couple to be encouraged not to have intercourse at all. Instead, they are given a series of assignments to do at home, in private. The first exercise usually instructs them to spend time touching each other in nonsexual ways. Eventually, they are told to take turns touching each other sensuously while the recipient describes what feels good and what doesn't.

At each session, the therapist notes how the exercises were done and whether the couple is interacting differently. Depending on what problem is being treated, new exercises are assigned. Most couples who experience sexual problems have difficulties talking about them to each other. Without input, they cannot know how to make things better. That's where sex therapy comes in. There is no standard course of treatment; some come for one session, others are seen weekly for years.

Sensate Focus Exercises

The term *sensate focus* is derived from Masters and Johnson, who wanted to get their couples to "focus their attention on the physical sensation." They found that many couples were too quick to try to have intercourse, and that they knew little about touching each other's bodies in ways that could be relaxing, exciting, and sensual. The object of the exercises is to take turns—that is, one person does the touching while the other is touched—and a central part is learning to talk with each other about what feels good and what does not. I suggest that couples try to see what new information they can discover about both their own and their partner's responses to touch.

Initially, the idea is to see what feels pleasurable; there is no demand to feel aroused sexually. This instruction in itself is often experienced as an enormous relief and reduces the pressure to "do it right."

Time needs to be set aside to do the exercises two or three times a week, and that in itself often presents a challenge. I encourage couples to think about what they have found promotes a comfortable atmosphere (e.g., music, low light, taking a bath or shower together).

The exercises include the following guidelines:

* Refrain from having intercourse (the idea is to reduce performance pressure).
* Take turns in who touches and who is touched.
* Be "selfish" when touched—focus all your attention on what the touch feels like and what you would like.
* Use touch that includes light stroking, massaging, kissing, licking, and caressing.
* Talk directly and explain what you enjoy or dislike.
* Shift the focus from *performance* to *pleasure and enjoyment*.

In most situations, intensive therapy to understand the "roots" of conflicts is not necessary. Often, a sexually oriented therapy can cure or significantly improve matters within weeks. For many, the therapist is the first person with whom they can have an open, nonjudgmental discussion about sexual matters.

The structured setting, in which tasks are broken down into their smallest components, almost immediately relieves the pressure. The specific assignments are often described by couples as enjoyable. There may be concern that the "exercises" are unspontaneous, but this is soon replaced by comfort in talking and doing things with each other physically that feel relaxing and comfortable. The climate is better for talking with each other, and couples are so relieved not to have to worry about the "grand performance" of intercourse. For many, it is the first time in years that they have spent any time caressing or touching each other's bodies while at the same time getting verbal feedback for what they are doing. It is helpful to change the direction of things and to have some successes on which to build. The regular meetings with the therapist provide some incentive for doing the homework assignments and a place to review the progress with some encouragement.

Couples With Problems—The How and Why of Treatment

*W*hen I treat couples, I try to form an outline in my mind that provides me with a map of the relationship. This includes learning about how the couple met, what drew them to each other, what the realities of their lives are, and what is not working well for them sexually. I may have an idea of what is needed in the therapy, but I have realized the need to keep an open mind about how to proceed. There are times when I may have to focus more on an interactional conflict before we can continue; I might need to pay attention to one partner's depression; or I might need to get additional gynecological or urological consultations. The course of treatment varies in length; I know some couples who have needed only one meeting and others who have required several years. I used to think that I could predict this, but I have learned that there are so many determinants that I now take a wait-and-see approach. The question of what actually happens in the therapy is an unknown for many couples seeking treatment. Following are the stories of some of the couples I have seen, what they told me, how I formulated the problem, and what we did during therapy. The following topics are addressed:

* Sexual difficulties
  - Inhibited sexual desire
  - Premature ejaculation
  - Infrequent sex
  - "Impotence" and "frigidity"
  - Vaginismus
  - Impotence
  - Low sexual desire and erectile difficulties
* A tale of two families—remarried with children
* Men, myths, and sex

Sexual Difficulties

Inhibited Sexual Desire

One of the more remarkable "cures" I've witnessed involved a man I saw whose complaint was low desire. He was in his late 30s and had been married for about 8 years. He had struggled for years with depression and had seen a number of therapists, none of whom seemed to have been very helpful. I could tell when I was questioning him that he resented the probing and was not happy that he was in my office. For him, it was a little like taking castor oil: unpleasant, but it might have some beneficial effects. I struggled to get through the interview; he was so reticent it felt as if I was pulling teeth to get any information from him.

Finally, in desperation, I asked whether there was anything that turned him on. He told me that he and his wife had gone to an X-rated film and after that had had great sex. He added that his wife did this willingly and clearly enjoyed the experience. It was as if a light bulb switched on for me, and I asked if he had a VCR.

(This was before the days of a VCR in every home.) The transformation in his facial expression was absolutely dramatic. He grinned from ear to ear and said, "I know what you're thinking!" Actually he did—I suggested that he rent some adult movies and see if this made a difference for him. We then got into an animated discussion about how many people needed to watch sexually explicit movies to help them feel freer to have a sexual imagination. I told him that if it did not work, to let me know. He left with a big smile and warm handshake.

About a half an hour later, I received a call from his wife who asked, "Did you really say that?" I told her I had, to which she replied, "But the man is depressed!" I agreed with her but added that it was clear that he had little use for therapy and resented any overture I made. She confirmed that the movie had been a success, and I suggested that they had nothing to lose. I heard from his internist about 6 months later that the sexual problem had resolved!

My providing an encouraging response was helpful to this man. Many people have trouble allowing themselves to have sexual fantasies, and the result is that they feel constricted and uncomfortable sexually. In not "forcing" him to endure this intrusive therapy, but instead supporting what had worked for him before, I could form a positive connection with this man that enabled him to "go it alone."

Premature Ejaculation

The treatment of premature ejaculation is usually relatively simple and straightforward. The success rate is about 90% in a relatively short time. However, there are situations where the sexual symptom is what keeps the relationship somewhat incomplete. This usually relates to trouble people may experience in recognizing dependency and attachments to their partners. As long as there is a sexual symptom, the relationship is less than perfect, and people are less prone to the conflicts around intimacy. It is in these more complex situations that the therapist has the opportunity to understand what is being expressed in the sexual symptom and to help the couple get beyond it.

Many years ago, I saw a couple whose identifying complaint was premature ejaculation. The couple stated quite directly that they did not want to have a talking therapy that would focus on their relationship; they had had oceans of individual therapy and couple's therapy and felt that they had an exquisite understanding of all their "neuroses." I try to respond to the stated complaint and see where that takes us. The couple had been married for about 16 years and had a solid relationship but had been troubled for years by the husband's difficulty in delaying ejaculation.

We started off with the sensate focus exercises, and the couple greeted the instruction to avoid any direct sexual stimulation with enormous relief. They described a new experience in learning how touch could be pleasurable and felt free of the anxiety that had been so entrenched around intercourse. I then added the "squeeze technique" exercise, where the wife would stimulate her husband's penis with her hand until orgasm was approaching. He would indicate that he was about to come, and she would then squeeze his penis at its base, which interrupts the orgasm reflex. The progress was striking. He was soon able to learn much better orgasmic control, and both were thrilled at the progress they were making.

The next step involved his putting his penis into her vagina and letting it rest there. The idea is to have the husband get used to the sensations of having his penis in his wife's vagina without any pressure to thrust or control orgasm. However, an unforeseen problem developed because I used the term *vaginal containment* to describe his keeping his penis in her vagina. (Early in my clinical career, I often used the terminology that had been developed by Masters and Johnson. When their book was written in the late 1950s, they were anxious that it be received as serious scientific study.)

The next week, I could tell as soon as I met the couple in the waiting room that this had been a bad week. They were quiet and looked miserable in contrast to the giggling and joviality of the past several sessions. As soon as I closed my office door the husband lamented that it had been a terrible week and that he had been unable to get an erection. "It all started when you talked about vaginal entrapment," he said. He then talked about his dread at trying intercourse and related a dream he had the night before. In his dream he came into the kitchen to feed a bird in a cage. He put his hand in to get the bird, but it flapped around in a panic and then keeled over dead, "all shriveled up" at the bottom of the cage.

The wife also had a dream taking place in the kitchen. In her dream, she entered the kitchen in time to see her child putting his hand into a food processor that was switched on. These dreams and the experience of being unable to get an erection changed the direction of the therapy dramatically. The couple was eager to understand the meaning behind this—and we were soon involved in a process to understand how each was terrified of feeling and expressing anger and how this was expressed in their sexual difficulty.

Although they had had much previous therapy, little in this regard had been explored. They each had critical, demeaning, and intrusive parents and had never dealt with this directly. Instead of feeling separate and independent from their parents, they did with each other what the parents had done with them, and sex became the arena in which anger and fear were played out. We spent several months discussing situations regarding each set of parents and various parental visits. Their understanding increased enormously, and they were both able to fend off parental criticisms appropriately and more clearly define their own relationship as distinct from their respective families.

After about 9 months of this, I asked about the sexual problems. They had on their own been practicing the exercises I had originally suggested, and the premature ejaculation had disappeared. I don't know what had not worked in their other therapies, but bringing together a variety of techniques that included initially some concrete suggestions for learning better ejaculatory control coupled with understanding the powerful influences of their parental experiences on their inner feelings enabled them to free themselves from the bonds of the past. They could then enter into a more open relationship that allowed them to apply and benefit from the sex therapy.

Often, apparently simple problems reveal hidden complexities after starting with the behavioral approach. I saw one man in his early 40s who had suffered premature ejaculation all his life. He had read the usual textbooks on the subject and had tried the recommendations on his own with little success. His adolescent sexual development was filled with one unfortunate setback after the next. Just as he discovered the pleasures of masturbation, he developed bladder problems that required many visits to a urologist and instruments inserted through his penis into his bladder. What had been a normal transition was suddenly colored by fear, exposure, embarrassment, and actual physical pain. There was so much anxiety associated with his penis that further sexual exploration was always associated with a worry that he might be doing something that would harm his genitals.

When he finally attempted to have intercourse, he ejaculated very quickly and felt humiliated. Early ejaculation is common when people first begin to have intercourse. However, with his backdrop of genital ailment, this was devastating. He experienced anxiety every time he contemplated sex. He finally did enter a relationship with a woman who was quite inexperienced and who was supportive and nonjudgmental. They married, and after several years of marriage, they finally sought help. The wife talked about her sexual inexperience and her wish that her husband would simply know what to do. She was somewhat hesitant to enter therapy, feeling that it was "his" problem. I might add that this is often the reaction of one partner. I try to point out that assigning fault or blame is not my role, but that seeing both partners allows me to address parts of the interaction I would not usually hear about if only one partner were there. What was interesting with this couple was that his premature ejaculation began to improve quite rapidly. Rather than greeting this with enthusiasm and relief, the wife began to withdraw and become distant and removed. She avoided sex and would instigate fights that would result in both feeling distant. The couple did notice the paradox in this behavior, and I tried to understand what it meant.

The wife had come from a divorced family and was terrified

that her marriage would also end in divorce. As long as the focus was on the husband's sexual difficulties, she could feel more comfortable with the idea that there was something wrong with him, and she had to put up with an incomplete relationship, about which she would complain. However, as things changed for him, she was confronted with a more complete relationship, and without realizing it, began to worry that she now had something that she valued and could potentially lose. Her withdrawal preempted the possible loss. The therapy is still in process. I hope that I can help her understand the fear of attachment and at the same time support her husband's feelings of sexual competence.

Infrequent Sex

The balance between attachment and the worry about loss is a fragile one for many, and the drama is often played out in marriage. The therapist needs to integrate an understanding of each partner's needs and personalities with the flow in the marriage and the way these themes get played out sexually. Things are not always what they appear to be. I had been seeing a couple who had been married for many years, and each was terrified of getting close and feeling too dependent on the other. A recurring complaint was they did not have sex frequently enough.

The wife came from an alcoholic family and felt she was responsible for everything in the marriage and that she deserved very little. The husband's family was aloof and distant, but his mother had developed a chronic illness when he was in his teens and he had to care for her. She died before he graduated high school. In the marriage, the two played out the seesaw of attachment and possible loss, each provoking the other to retreat just enough to let the fears diminish but not so far as to be overwhelming. The couple had been doing quite well, and we had begun to retrace the patterns in each family. They went out alone one evening and had a good time with each other, actually feeling warm and affectionate. They each entertained ideas of making love upon their return. When they entered the bedroom, the husband said, "Why do you always have to leave things such a mess—you really are a pig!" to which the wife angrily replied, "I'm a mess? Have you seen the bathroom with all your stuff on the floor?"

The two stalked into separate rooms, and the romance was gone. For them, making love was associated with too much closeness. They had had to create some distance: the husband by picking the fight and the wife by reacting accordingly. I helped them in getting a handle on this process, so that now if one is provocative, the other is able to be less reactive and asks, "Are you trying to retreat from being close?"

"Impotence" and "Frigidity"

I witnessed a particularly surprising outcome with a couple in their late 30s who had been married for about 15 years. The first time they came into my office, the wife sat down and announced that she was frigid and her husband was impotent! When I explored their relationship, the marriage seemed rigid and inflexible. The wife came across as controlling, demeaning, and angry, and the husband appeared frightened and passive. There was a long-standing pattern of his deferring to her, and they avoided talking about much. Sex had never been particularly rewarding, and for the past 8 years, the husband had been unable to get an erection at all. They had decided to seek therapy because the wife worked as a supervisor in a large office and her female employees (all in their early 20s) saw her as a parent figure with whom they could discuss their problems. They would talk with her about their boyfriends and their sexual relationships, and she began to feel that there was something that she was missing in her marriage.

There seemed to be such a fixed inflexibility in their relationship that I worried that therapy—particularly sex therapy—would be of little use. I thought that there were long-standing, difficult "character issues" that were not going to change easily and suggested that they think carefully about whether they wanted to embark on this course of therapy. In essence, I suggested that they might not want to rock the boat. They called back about a week later saying that they did want to go ahead with the program. With some trepidation I agreed, and we started some discussions about their sexual feelings. I initially suggested the touching exercises where there was no pressure to become aroused. They did reasonably well with them, but the wife then said that she did not know what it was to feel aroused. As we talked more, it was clear that, although they had had intercourse over the years, she had never felt aroused sexually, and the idea of being "turned on" was quite foreign to her.

I was relatively new at doing this when I saw them, and I had read that electric vibrators were helpful for women whose sexual feelings were blocked. I gingerly raised the idea that she might like to consider trying the use of a (and then had a hard time getting the word out) vibrator. I expected her to be outraged and to threaten reporting me to the Board of Registration in Medicine for lewd and lascivious suggestions. To my surprise, she eagerly embraced the idea and said, "If you think it will help, I want to try it." When I saw them the following week, they had been on a citywide search for a vibrator and had been unable to locate one. We finally tracked one down in the health care section of a department store.

When they came in to their next session, the wife was quite enthusiastic. She had used the vibrator and was excited by the enjoyable sexual feelings she experienced. "Now I don't need my husband," she joked, and we all laughed. (This was a hostile and demeaning remark, but it was important to let it stand as a "joke" because I wanted to reinforce her good feelings about discovering her sexual responses.) They continued to do the exercises faithfully, and each week we would add another "building block." Eight weeks after starting the therapy, they were having intercourse on a fairly regular basis and enjoying it. This was one of the defining moments for me because it clearly demonstrated how, in the presence of what I had determined was a rigid, fixed situation, this couple had moved rapidly to change a pattern in a gratifying way.

Vaginismus

Many therapists still support the idea that resolving earlier conflicts is a prerequisite to changing sexual behavior. Despite
absolutely miserable therapeutic results, it continues to be a
recommended approach.

With one couple, the woman suffered from a moderately severe
form of vaginismus. Intercourse was possible but always extremely
painful. Her boyfriend was a sensitive guy who could not tolerate
producing pain when they made love. The interesting fact was that
she enjoyed being aroused sexually and was able to have an orgasm
with manual stimulation of her genitals.

She sought therapy to deal with the difficulty, and there was a
gold mine of material to be explored. She had a variety of recollections of events when she was 7 or 8 years old that pointed to a
possibility that she might have been sexually abused. She recalled
being seen by a doctor for a routine exam as a child and feeling
terrified about being in the examining room with him alone. Her
therapist tried to engage her in recalling the memories, with the
expectation that some recollection of abuse would surface and that
a process of healing would follow its discovery. However, nothing
worked, and the therapy reached an impasse after several years.

I attempted initially to work with the couple using the graded
touching exercises I have previously described. There were some
changes, but nothing dramatic. I then showed the couple a teaching
video called *Treating Vaginismus*, discussed the relaxation techniques described, and suggested that she view the film at home,
experiment with the relaxation techniques, and begin to use some
vaginal dilators. Having her partner involved was very helpful. He
genuinely supported her and was interested in learning how he could
help. Initially, she practiced the relaxation exercises on her own,
and then included him as they began together to try to insert vaginal
dilators of varying size into her vagina. Although she dreaded doing
this, much to her surprise, she had no pain, and her relief spurred her
on to try the larger dilators. Soon she was able to have intercourse
comfortably, though she often worried that pain would occur.

In this instance, a combination approach really made the difference. She tried specific exercises, her boyfriend was involved in the treatment, they had a place where they felt safe in talking directly about what was happening, and they saw some results quickly. There is tremendous value in providing a "benevolent parent" model. Helping a couple have pleasurable sexual experiences enables them to draw on their own resources to rapidly acquire skills and techniques. This is somewhat like the role of a coach in sports: The coach helps the individual get in touch with specific strengths and abilities, identifies what needs practice and correcting, and devises drills and exercises to enhance skills. Usually, the individual has a positive relationship with the coach that can bring out previously unrecognized strengths.

Impotence

Impotence affects about 10% of men and is the source of considerable pain and suffering. These men suffer shame, low self-esteem, and anxiety at every sexual encounter. The idea of fun and pleasure in sex disappears. This leads to a reinforcing cycle of failures. Usually, their partners feel confused and worry that they may somehow be part of the cause. Social situations where sexual jokes are traded become excruciating, and the quality of the relationship declines. As I have mentioned earlier, there are both psychological and medical causes of impotence, which overlap in many situations. It's difficult to sort them out and offer an appropriate treatment. Our understanding of the physical mechanisms of erectile functioning is still rudimentary. We have many fancy terms to describe the process that would suggest that our sophistication is greater than it is.

A few years ago, I saw a couple who were in their early 30s. They had been married for about 8 years and were eager to have children. The problem was that the husband could not maintain an erection. They would begin to make love, and he would feel aroused and get an erection. However, as soon as they would begin to have intercourse, his erection would disappear. They were extremely depressed and could not understand what they were doing wrong.

I met with the husband alone to take a more detailed history. He was a tall, attractive man who was successful in his profession. He had experimented sexually in his teens and had never had any difficulty maintaining erections. He was comfortable with sex and enjoyed sharing his feelings with women. In his early 20s, he had been involved in a long-term relationship, and sex had been just fine. As the relationship began to fall apart after about 3 years, he noticed that occasionally he would lose his erection. He did not pay much attention to this, thinking that it was probably a function of the breakdown of the relationship (this phenomenon is quite common in such situations).

He then met his wife, but noticed that from the start, he would lose his erection. He could not understand this, as he felt very excited with her and had never previously questioned his sexuality. Several years ago, I would have thought that there was a psychological problem here. This situation met some of the criteria that the early work of Masters and Johnson and Helen Singer Kaplan established. One could make a case for the development of a repeated cycle of performance anxiety. (Therapists love to formulate their patients' problems and translate them into neat hypotheses. Over the years, I have come to realize how far from the truth we often are, and feel that my hunches are simply that—and it's up to me to prove them.) In this man's history, something simply did not fit. He had been perfectly comfortable with sex during his teens, had masturbated with regularity and comfort, had had several enjoyable sexual relationships, and had also integrated his sexuality with the development of a close and intense long-term relationship. After the first relationship ended, he formed a close and intimate bond with the woman who was to become his wife. They were warm and loving with each other; she was supportive and compassionate and did not feel either angry or self-doubting about his difficulties.

This was around the time that a urology group in Boston (Drs. Krane and Goldstein) had developed the concept of "failure to fill."

In their studies, they found that many men had experienced some pelvic trauma such as falling onto the crossbar of a bicycle, gymnastic injuries where there had been injuries to their perineum (the area between anus and scrotum), or being kicked in the groin. They found that this led in some situations to damage of the pelvic blood vessels so that the valves were unable to hold the pressure necessary to maintain an erection. The men could get an erection, but as soon as they would attempt intercourse and thrusting (which applied force to the penis) the blood was literally squeezed out of the penis. (The usual systolic blood pressure for men is around 130 mm of mercury. The pressure required to maintain an erection is over 400 mm of mercury. With damaged valves, it was not possible to keep the pressure high enough.)

The recommendation for this couple was a trial of intrapenile injections, which resulted in a sustained erection. The couple was delighted with the results, and treatment ended. About a year later, I received a birth announcement. The pleasure for the therapist (in conjunction with the urological help) in making such a difference to two people's live is wonderful. I have often reflected on a few patients I had seen more than 10 years ago, who, I now realize, had venous leak syndrome. I had approached them from the psychological perspective with obviously little improvement.

Increasingly, we are seeing men who have impotence problems with no identifiable cause. If they have had satisfactory sexual relationships before the change, I am loath to view the difficulty as psychological and am more inclined to think that at this point our diagnostic sophistication is a limiting factor.

Low Sexual Desire and Erectile Difficulties

The balance necessary for a good sex life is easily disrupted for many people, and without a supportive place to discuss what is not working right, the problem can grow and assume a life of its own, becoming woven into the fabric of the relationship. I was asked to consult with one couple in their early 50s. The husband had low sexual desire and a persistent inability to maintain an erection. They had been married for nearly 20 years and had successfully raised three children, who were all doing well. They described their relationship as good, although they had always felt tension around sex, which increased as the children began to leave home.

Both of them had had many years of individual therapy; the wife had sought treatment for some anxiety and depression and felt very good about the outcome. Over the years, the husband had consulted several therapists in an attempt to overcome his sexual difficulties but with little long-term effect. I was a little skeptical myself about what I could do. The husband was a pleasant man but was extremely obsessional and not close to his feelings. I talked with him more on his own and learned that he functioned extremely well in his business but was reluctant to confront people directly and seemed to be uncomfortable seeing himself as competent. I hypothesized to myself that the sexual difficulty was an expression of his conflict around competence and assertiveness, but wondered—considering all the therapy he had over the years—what I would have to offer.

The wife talked about how she felt angry much of the time and realized that her overreactions were related to her sexual frustration. She tried to be understanding, but it was wearing a little thin. I spent weeks trying to learn more about their day-to-day interactions and quickly learned that, although the wife expressed her anger directly, he kept his quite hidden, saying that he "did not have an angry bone in his body." Without making any interpretation to him about my ideas that he had trouble being assertive, I suggested that over the ensuing week he take notes on anything that was the least bit irritating to him regarding his wife. The next week, he came in with a long list of items—most of which are the usual trivia that couples struggle over, such as squeezing the toothpaste in the middle of the tube or leaving hairs in the sink. The wife responded with surprise and encouragement, saying that unless he told her these things, she had no way of knowing what irritated him, nor could she modify her behavior.

After this assignment, things seemed to ease up between the

two of them, and I introduced the touching exercises. I suggested that they take turns touching each other's bodies, talking about what they liked and what they did not like but not focusing on producing any sexual arousal. Many couples initially react unfavorably to these instructions because they seem nonspontaneous, forced, and boring. Sometimes they are; but most couples come to feel less tense and are freed to experience something with each other that is new and enjoyable. The key, in my view, is helping couples talk with each other directly about likes and dislikes, because they usually have had little success in doing that comfortably.

The touching exercises went surprisingly well; the wife felt that they were doing something different that offered potential for change, and the husband enjoyed the idea of following instructions and completing a task. However, I was careful to pay attention to the husband's hidden agenda of not feeling comfortable in confronting his wife in other areas. My theory was that if there were unaddressed items that he did not deal with directly, they would go underground and be expressed through his inability to maintain an erection. The exercises continued to go well, and I gradually added new assignments that included genital caressing. Both of them experienced pleasure and enjoyment, and the husband began to feel more confident.

In one telling encounter, the couple had gone away for a weekend trip, and before leaving to come home, the husband had wanted to make some coffee. The wife said they did not have time and urged the husband to get in the car so that they could leave. As they were driving, he realized that he felt angry and stopped at a doughnut shop. In the store, he told his wife that he was angry that she would not let him have the coffee. She said that she did not realize that it was that important to him and apologized for her insistent tone—and that was the end of it. They both let it go and moved on. For the husband, it was a series of important steps: He initially identified his wish (wanting coffee), he realized that he was not helpless and could have an impact on what he wanted, and he not only recognized his annoyance with his wife but told her. All of this may seem simple, but it represented a significant change in how he dealt with his wife. In the past, he would have held all this in, not knowing that he was frustrated and angry, and would have withdrawn in a variety of ways, including sexually.

I have mentioned that in the early stages of the sexual exercises, couples are urged not to attempt intercourse at all. This takes performance pressure out of the situation and helps them direct their attention to pleasure and enjoyment. However, the couple came in one time and reported with a great deal of satisfaction that things had been going so well in one of their exercise sessions that they had decided to disregard the instructions. They had intercourse, felt relaxed, and enjoyed the experience. I was delighted and encouraged by the husband's newfound assertiveness. After 9 weeks, the couple stopped the treatment. I have to admit that I was surprised at how quickly there had been a turnaround. I heard from the couple about 6 months later, and they had continued to make progress. They had taken a vacation together and said that it was the best ever.

Over the years, I wondered whether the changes had been sustained, but I felt that no news was probably good news. Then about 5 years later, they again called, and the erectile difficulties had returned. When I saw them, it became apparent that the husband was suffering depression. He was about to retire, and things had not worked out as well as he had hoped with his business. He was worried about their finances and realized that he would have to scale back their financial expectations. He felt that he had let his wife down and felt a huge burden on his shoulders. In this instance, the sexual exercises were not going to be useful. I have often seen men whose initial complaint is impotence but who have an unrecognized depression. Their penises become the marker for their sad feelings.

The approach I took this time was threefold: 1) I prescribed an antidepressant for the husband, 2) I helped the two talk directly about the financial situation and helped them go over the details, and 3) I suggested they consult with a financial planner. This way, they would have some outside professional advice that they would pursue together, and the husband would not feel that it was his sole responsibility. The wife liked the idea of learning more about their finances. Over the next 6 months we met regularly. They set up a clear financial plan for themselves, the husband became more optimistic, and his sexual functioning returned.

Their story is not unusual and is a good example of the ebb and flow of sex and relationships over time. This couple had over the years formed a committed bond with each other, although they had been unable to deal with the sexual difficulties. They finally were able to seek out an appropriately focused treatment and master their sexual problems. (For many older couples, there were no treatments available when they were in their 20s.) Finally, the husband's changed circumstances and resulting depression affected his sexual capacity, and they returned for a different kind of treatment. This helped them use their own considerable resources to overcome their current problems.

A Tale of Two Families: Remarried With Children

Divorce and remarriage are with us to stay. The complexity of breaking up, keeping connections with ex-spouses and children, and then remarrying and having a mixture of old and new families is often daunting. Couples have to balance the loyalties and disappointments of the past with the excitement and challenges of the new relationship. People often worry about the possibility of another failure, and they may blow any disagreement or disappointment out of proportion as a signal of failure. Often there are adolescent children, and this brings special challenges. The adolescents are usually just beginning to have sexual feelings, and the discomfort for them in being around "newly marrieds" who may be intensely sexual creates a particularly delicate tension.

This was not the issue, though, with Drew and Ellen (not their real names), a couple I consulted with who had been divorced many years before meeting each other and who both had children from their prior marriages. They had known each other for many years, renewed their friendship, and began to develop a relationship. Initially, they were excited to have found each other again, loved the process of sharing their lives together, and had great sex. They decided to get married, but soon after the wedding, sex became the wheel that squeaked. Ellen found that her sexual interest diminished and that she almost had an aversion to being sexual, which resulted in tensions and fights. Frightened that another relationship was going to fail, they sought therapy.

Ellen's mother had been very controlling and critical and even now would call her and assault her with a list of her failures. Drew, on the other hand, described his family as warm and caring, a model of warmth in sharp contrast to Ellen's. So initially, I had a clear sense of the difficulty for Ellen, but Drew's family was something of a mystery. The couple did not realize that the idea of a relationship being "complete" was scary. Neither of them had experienced being in a long-term relationship that continued to feel good; they both described the relentless feeling of decay that set into their previous marriages and how they felt powerless to affect any change. Gradually, each had become conditioned to believing that a relationship with another individual would ultimately be unsatisfying, and they did not realize how they literally had to keep one part "missing" for the relationship to feel familiar.

Almost invariably, couples reenact family patterns—though they have very little awareness of doing so. Keeping the patterns familiar makes them feel as if they had never left "home," and therefore they never have to deal with the sadness of letting go. With Ellen and Drew, the struggle over sex continued with considerable force, and Drew felt cheated and betrayed. In his view, Ellen had been transformed from the woman he had gotten to know, and he talked endlessly about her "difficulties." He did not notice how he was afraid of being alone and how much he would use sex as a way to feel good and whole. (I have noticed that men often talk about how they feel good about themselves if they have sex, whereas women focus more on the meaning of the relationship and the ways they feel noticed and understood.) I noticed that when

Drew was less urgent and pressuring, they enjoyed sex and felt close. There were many therapy sessions that ended with Ellen feeling angry and Drew depressed and hopeless.

Gradually, the relationship began to heal, and they reached a new level of stability. They found a way of talking to each other that emphasized telling each other what they were feeling. This made it much easier for them to be compassionate rather than repeating the escalating cycle of recriminations and withdrawals.

I have seen this pattern with several couples who have divorced and then remarried in their late 40s, and I have identified common characteristics and developed a theory about what happens.

Marital tension is expressed in a diminished sexual interest that confuses the couple and results in each partner's feeling hurt and angry. Many couples who married in their early 20s inadvertently short-circuited some of the developmental tasks relating to separating from their original family and defining who they are. They get married and have little idea about what a give-and-take relationship involves, but they are sustained by the novelty of feeling independent. Often, they have children soon and are then confined to pursuing a path in which they deal with jobs and careers, children and schools, and the whole gamut of family "stuff" that is engaging and preoccupying.

Gradually, a feeling of emptiness begins to surface that, if powerful enough, may result in divorce. So at age 40-something, people are thrust into the "dating scene" with a feeling of confusion and disorientation. Society views them as adults (they may be quite accomplished professionally, have children, and look like grownups), but when it comes to being in a relationship, they feel like adolescents. In adolescence, they may not have formed strong attachments outside the family where they could learn to identify characteristics that they liked and disliked. Now, however, they have the life experiences to know better what is important in a relationship and may make a good choice of partner on that basis.

But they have not dealt with the delicate balance in human relationships stirred by intensely close, dependent feelings. They want to be involved with a loving partner whom they in turn can love, but their life experiences have been so colored by disappointment that they unwittingly reinforce the other patterns that screen out those interactions that could lead to closer connections. I believe that in these situations it is crucial to understand what was unsatisfying in the original family of each partner. As long as one or the other (or both) clings to a sanitized view of the parents, they are almost compelled to repeat the patterns in the current relationship.

I don't believe, however, that one should go on a psychological crusade to vilify parents as awful people. They usually did their best and tried to be good parents. What is important is to recognize the patterns and disappointments that almost invariably exist with parents. I try to explain this idea to couples as the "hopelessness of childhood" and the "hopefulness of couplehood." As a child, even if you were able to identify disappointments with your parents, you usually could not change much. This results in a sense that in a relationship it is hopeless to believe that needs can be met.

However, in a relationship between couples, there is the potential for each to listen and understand what the other wants and to respond reciprocally. Once a couple grasps the concept that they can be on the same team, they can relate to each other with totally surprising results. When the relational difficulties are not clearly identified, they often get channeled into the sexual arena and are expressed as lowered interest and desire. For remarried couples, being helped to integrate these complex issues and feel satisfaction and comfort is relieving and rewarding.

*M*en, *Myths, and Sex*

Over the past 20 years, our understanding of the emotional concerns of women has broadened. It is only recently that attention has been directed to understanding the ways men feel vulnerable. The stereotype is of men *doing* rather than feeling. In the realm of sexuality, men are often thought of as "having only one thing on their minds." Concerns about being sexually incompetent are much more common than has been recognized. I have seen three young men in the past year for whom this was a major problem.

Josh (not his real name) was 19 when he first came to see me, plagued by the fact that he had never been able to maintain an erection with a partner. He was very down on himself and convinced that he was the first person to be so afflicted. He was genuinely surprised to learn that erectile difficulties are very common, particularly when people first begin to be sexually active.

Josh's father was an aggressive businessman who was demanding and very critical, often pointing out Josh's failings. When I first saw Josh, he described dreading asking a woman for a date and was totally preoccupied with feeling humiliated. Although Josh initially focused on sex, it was his relationship with his father that gave him trouble. When he was on a date, it was as if his father was telling him he was going to fail.

My explanations made sense for him, and with my encouragement he began to date. I urged him to get to know the person and see whether he liked her before feeling the need to be sexual. This was an enormous relief for him. I have found that many men have the mistaken idea (reinforced in no small measure by television, movies, and books) that the manly thing to do is to have sex on the first or second date. Josh was relieved to know that he could take his time. He also realized that in his previous dating, he had barely known the person he was with and had no way of feeling trusting enough to express his vulnerability and uncertainty. As he understood this more, and with encouragement in therapy, Josh was able to trust his partner with his concerns. Much to his surprise, when he did talk about his uncertainty, she was understanding and helpful, and his erectile difficulties disappeared. I was able to act as a counterbalance to his negative, critical father, and I helped him see his partner as a trusting collaborator. In that setting, he was able to put aside the intense worry about not measuring up to the standards set by his dad.

Barry (again, not his real name) was 29 when he sought help. He was a single professional who had not dated much but was now in a relationship with a woman he really loved. His problem was that he was not able to have an orgasm with her. He felt desire, felt aroused, could have intercourse, but an orgasm seemed impossible. He too was filled with shame and embarrassment, and he was surprised to learn that other men suffered with this problem. He had little opportunity to get much sexual information from either parents or teachers. He masturbated a bit, but felt guilty, and worried that it would make his problem worse. Barry was eager for information about sexual responses, and once I started to provide him answers, his questions and curiosity grew. I reassured him about masturbation and told him that most men masturbated throughout life. I suggested that rather than inhibiting his sexual activity, it might help him get more in touch with his own erotic feelings.

Within 2 weeks, Barry was "cured." It took a little support and encouragement for him to have his first orgasm with his girlfriend, and thereafter he did fine. The main problem was that he was struggling in the dark with no information, and feeling that he did not know what he was doing. In addition, I realized that he had mixed feelings about expressing openly his sexual interests. My role was to help him draw on his inner feelings and facilitate his getting in touch with his own strengths. The role of coach again comes to mind.

One of the most surprising problems I encountered was a young professional couple, David and Chris (not their real names), who had been married for 6 years and had *never* had intercourse with each other. David was afraid to get undressed in front of Chris or to have her touch his body. Somehow, they entered into a conspiracy of silence, and the relationship simply went along without sex. Using a modification of Masters and Johnson's directive approach, I gave them some touching exercises to try at home. We met weekly to review progress, answer questions, and provide support. We worked out ways they could initially start touching each other with clothes on and thereby lessen David's fear.

I was repeatedly struck by my own stereotypical responses. I reflexively thought that it was odd that David did not welcome

Chris's advances and felt so uncomfortable with her touch. He had been involved in a lengthy individual therapy, and I noticed that he and his therapist seemed stuck over concerns that he was homosexual. Although David and his therapist had spent years talking about this, nothing seemed to get better in David's marriage. I determined that David and Chris really liked one another, were committed, and were genuinely pained about not being able to consummate their marriage. They felt that they were strange and weird, and they were terrified that friends might somehow find out their secret. I found that I had to improvise as we went along. David and Chris made rapid progress, and the touching exercises became more open, less fraught with worry, and more enjoyable. Within 6 weeks, they had consummated their marriage. The change in their overall appearance (facial expression and general demeanor) was testament to the dramatic changes that had taken place in their relationship.

Many men experience great conflict over what they perceive as societal expectations to act as "real, sexually aggressive men" and their own feelings of ignorance and incompetence. The penis is extremely susceptible to failure in the face of emotional stress. Men and women alike need to talk more about what they don't know, what they fear, and what they share.

Chapter 9

The Family

*T*he American family has been under siege, with many social, economic, and political forces exerting tremendous pressures on this institution. In its healthy and well-functioning state, the family has enormous force and power. It provides the framework for nurturing and growth and helps lay the foundation for the future generation. When a couple makes the decision to become a family by having a child, they embark on a journey filled with unexpected challenges, rewards, and disappointments. Each of these experiences in turn may have an impact on a couple's sexual relationship, as the questions presented in this chapter illustrate. As children grow, parents are put in the sometimes uncomfortable position of needing to provide sexual education and guidance. This chapter will encourage you to think about your own values—where you stand and how you believe your children should conduct themselves as they become sexual.

The following topics are addressed:

* Pregnancy and Birth
    - His sperm won't meet my egg
    - He wants a child!
    - Jogging and fertility
    - Husbands and pregnancy—is there "womb envy"?

-   Low sexual desire after child is born
-   Vaginal changes with childbirth

✳ Children, Sex, and Parents—Can We Talk?
-   Talking to your kids about sex
-   Erections and infants
-   Sex with kids in the room
-   Children bathing together
-   Nudity and your children
-   Playing doctor
-   Sexual harassment at 12?

✳ Teens and Sex
-   Puberty changes
-   Helping kids to wait
-   A 15-year-old keeping score
-   Mutual masturbation among teens
-   How common is masturbation in adolescence?
-   Should masturbation be encouraged?
-   Parents' values and teens' sexual activities
-   Teens and AIDS
-   Is my son gay?
-   What causes a child to become a lesbian or homosexual adult?

*P*regnancy and Birth

The decision to have children represents a new phase in a couple's relationship. Some couples plan very carefully the exact time that they will attempt to conceive, others have a laid-back attitude about timing, and still others opt out of active decision making and suddenly find themselves with a child. For most couples, the transition is not accompanied by much difficulty. However, there are several potential pitfalls that may make the course a little rocky.

Couples may not anticipate the changes that occur both physically and emotionally during the pregnancy. The responsibility and changing roles may change the "feel" of the relationship in a way that was not anticipated. This may have unexpected effects on the sexual relationship.

Once the baby is born, the excitement, newness, and in many instances sheer exhaustion transform the marriage. No longer is the couple free to do what they please. The responsibility for the newborn child seems endless, and the impact on sexual feelings may be profound.

While most couples conceive without much difficulty, infertility may be a devastating problem. Couples who are having trouble conceiving may feel enormous disappointment, worry, pressure from families, shame about not conceiving, and a shift in viewing sex as a "natural" event to a complicated series of medical procedures. Sex under these circumstances is usually negatively affected with pain and stress.

> After 4 years of trying, I have not been able to conceive. A doctor has said my husband has a low sperm count, but he has two children from a previous marriage. I also have two children. What should we do?

Let me answer your question in two parts: It sounds as if you need to consult an infertility specialist. That you both have children is encouraging. The low sperm count by itself doesn't mean you can't have children. Sometimes, there may be a chemical "incompatibility"—the sperm, for whatever reason, may be less active in your vagina. Your doctor can perform a few routine tests, including a postcoital examination of sperm activity, to see if there are any readily identifiable causes.

Having addressed your question, let me add that the emotional impact of infertility on a couple is enormous, and often not addressed. The following issues contribute to the emotional stress associated with infertility:

* Both partners begin to focus on whether the wife gets her period, with pressure and tension mounting each month. After a

while, they may not even talk about it, but the worry is ever present, and mood swings associated with the waiting can be extreme.

＊ They may begin to obsess about why they cannot do what "everyone else seems to have no trouble with" and feel that they are defective. Often they do not openly express this, and each secretly harbors some notion of what is wrong with one or the other or both.

＊ Sex is no longer a source of pleasure and closeness but is closer to "work," as they try to have intercourse exactly at the right time. Intercourse becomes a means to an end rather than a mutually pleasurable act.

Needless to say, these negative emotional effects can greatly strain a couple's relationship. Often some support—whether it be from friends who have had similar difficulties, a counselor, or a therapy group—can make the experience easier to bear.

> **We've been married for about a year, and my husband is desperate for me to become pregnant. I had hoped that we would wait a few years to build some savings and allow me to advance in my job. Now I find that my desire for sex has plummeted. What can we do?**

It appears that you and your husband have inadvertently landed in a power struggle. He wants to have a child now, and you want to wait. This has created tension in your relationship, so it really is no surprise that your sexual desire has diminished. The sexual relationship has become the place where you are playing out this struggle. Sometimes, if the wife wants to have children and the husband does not, he may be uninterested in sex or even become impotent.

The two of you need to talk about your differing expectations and needs. Initiating a conversation may seem very difficult; you might start by saying, "I know I've been uninterested in sex lately. I think that's because I feel so pressured about getting pregnant. Can we talk about this?" This should open a discussion in which you can both express your positions and be clearer about where each of you stands. Why does he want to have children now? What makes it hard for him to wait? And why do you want to delay starting a family? If such a conversation creates too much tension, talk it out together with a professional who can help you work out a compromise.

> I'm 28 and want to start a family. I'm also a jogger who runs about 10 miles a day. I've heard that running makes it harder for a woman to conceive. Should I cut back on jogging or give it up while trying to get pregnant?

Exercise is extremely important for health and well-being but, done to excess, can have undesirable side effects. Some women who exercise a great deal *do* undergo a change in their hormonal system that may suppress ovulation.

If your periods have always been regular, and that has not changed since you took up jogging, there probably is no reason to change your pattern. However, if you've noticed any irregularity in your cycle, or if your periods have stopped altogether, cut back on your jogging and consult your gynecologist.

> Can a man be affected physically by his wife's pregnancy? My husband seemed to mimic my symptoms, from nausea to weight gain.

Yes, there are many reports of men who experience physical ailments associated with pregnancy while their wives are pregnant. By mimicking your experience, your husband is able to share it.

Keep in mind that pregnancy is usually a very intense time for a couple. There are significant role shifts as the two realize that they are about to become parents, and that this will create irrevocable changes in their lives. It sounds as if your husband identifies strongly with your physical changes. It may help to ask if he has noticed the degree to which his experiences are similar to yours, but I don't believe there is cause for alarm. Your husband certainly does not think that *he* is the one who is pregnant. John Nelson, a psychiatrist with whom I worked, coined the term "womb envy" to refer to unrecognized sadness many men feel from being unable to have the experience their wives do in carrying a baby.

Our first child is 3 months old. I haven't wanted sex since she was born and my husband is getting frustrated. Help!

Give yourself a break! Having a child is a major, life-altering event. You are no longer someone's child but have become someone's parent. First-time parents are often struck by the change they have brought into their lives; they have total responsibility for someone who is absolutely dependent and helpless. Gone are the carefree weekends, the leisurely dinners, and the late nights. In their place is an infant who is often very noisy at one end and seemingly very busy at the other!

Besides the great emotional changes (and the physical wear and tear of labor and delivery), you probably are exhausted. This is definitely not the time sexual feelings run high. Somehow you are going to have to let your husband know about the differences in your experiences. Usually, couples need several months—sometimes a year—to sort out the impact of parenthood and resume the kind of sexual relationship they had before the baby arrived. I have encountered husbands who have elicited awful guilt in their wives, talking about built-up sexual tension that is not being relieved. I'm afraid I don't have too much sympathy, and I would suggest that they consider other forms of release. Husbands should be able to share in the joy, excitement, and utter exhaustion of having created a new human being.

After having three children by natural childbirth, I don't enjoy sex anymore. I feel too "roomy." My doctor says this is normal, but it can't be. I actually don't feel anything during sex. Is there help for us?

During childbirth, all muscles and ligaments in the pelvis stretch to some degree. Many women have an episiotomy, in which the obstetrician cuts the vagina to ease the delivery. With most women, the vagina regains its elasticity and shape, although this may not always be the case. It sounds as if your vagina has not returned to its prepregnancy shape. What's important is that it feels different to you.

I suggest that you get a second opinion to evaluate the changes that may have occurred in your pelvis. In some cases, surgery is recommended to "tighten" the vagina, though I encourage you to ask the doctor many questions about what this involves. You may prefer to try nonsurgical possibilities, such as Kegel exercises. They increase the tone of the pelvic muscles and are simple to do. Imagine that you are urinating and want to stop the urine stream. The muscles you use are called the pubococcygeus (or PC) muscles. By contracting and relaxing these muscles several times each day, you may enhance your muscle tone. That will help you to "grasp" the penis when it is in your vagina.

It might be helpful to experiment with different positions for intercourse; some give the sensation of increased pressure and friction. Your husband might vary his thrusting, concentrating on a more shallow movement with the head of his penis closer to the opening of your vagina. This will provide increased stimulation to both of you.

Children, Sex, and Parents—Can We Talk?

I am often asked about how to talk to children about sex. However much theoretical advice they may read, this topic remains a source of discomfort for most parents. In part, I think that the difficulty has to do with the fact that many parents had little help or advice about sex from their own parents and thus did not have a role model for talking about the subject. In addition, discussing sex may get people in touch with some uncomfortable feelings that contribute to their feeling tongue-tied and awkward.

It is useful to reflect on your own experiences as a child, including where you learned about sex and from whom. In addition, think about what might have been helpful to you and at what age. The point is to try to use your own experiences to develop a method that will feel comfortable. Often, couples have not discussed much together about their own experiences, and the sharing is often revealing and helpful and can pave the way to talking with their children.

Frequently, adults seek advice about how to approach this subject when their children are almost in their teens. By this time, kids have usually acquired much information from their friends or older siblings and are usually unreceptive to any discussion about sex with their parents. I have noticed that fathers will often avoid the subject entirely and "leave it to the wife" to talk with the kids. Many wives feel that they are not able to be as helpful to their sons as they are able to be to their daughters, and they wish that their husbands could share the responsibility.

When it comes to deciding how much information is required, let kids tell you what they want to know and keep your answers simple, direct, and honest. Often, parents think in a complex, sophisticated way and try to give their children all the facts at once. Frankly, the kids don't want all the information, and furthermore they cannot integrate it.

Rather than planning a time when you will sit down with your kids to "talk seriously about sex," use family time together where the subject may come up without any planning. The car proves to be a wonderful place to have all sorts of discussions. The family is together, there is no television, and no one can leave. You can bring up the topic of puberty well before your child starts to develop sexually. Talking about the changes that will take place in their bodies gives children the information they need to be prepared when it begins to happen.

How do you communicate with children about sex?

I suggest giving your children reliable, reassuring information about their bodies, how reproduction takes place, and the value of emotional bonds before physical ones. When talking about body parts, use words such as *vagina* and *penis* rather than nicknames like "wee-wee," "peter," or "privates," which convey the idea that talking about sex is silly or embarrassing.

Everyone is bound to make some mistakes. I once mistakenly assumed that I needed to provide lots of facts for every question. I remember the jolt of panic I felt when one of my children asked me, "Where did I come from?" I was well into a discussion of egg and sperm before she interrupted me to say, "No. No. Was I born in Boston or Brookline?"

A guiding principle is to let your children tell you what they want to know and to keep your answers simple, direct, and honest. I believe that approach will give kids a good feeling about their bodies and help them see their bodies as a source of pleasure not only in the sexual realm but also in the sense that comes from being fit and self-confident.

My hope is that through talking and discussion, children will learn that sex is something that's best as a shared experience with someone they love and respect. I think that it is preferable for them to wait until they are young adults to become sexually active. Realistically, parents cannot control that. What's most important is that children's sexual activity not be conducted in ignorance or in a way that leads them to take serious health risks. These are hazardous times and there are dangers. It's up to parents to provide some sort of foundation for their children.

> While changing my infant son's diaper, I noticed, with great surprise, what I am sure was an erection. Is this possible? When do children become sexual persons?

You have made the important observation that arousal (at least if we measure it by erection) takes place very early on. One can assume that similar reactions take place with girls, although you can't see the immediate, outward evidence. From studies of adult sexual physiology, however, we know that engorgement of vaginal blood vessels is the counterpart to the blood vessels in the penis filling up.

Initially, children discover their genitals in a random way. They may inadvertently touch the penis or clitoris, be aware of an enjoyable feeling, and learn that this is something they can do repeatedly. Most parents have observed that children begin to touch their genitals quite early. As your children get older, you will want to communicate to them that privacy is an important component of touching their genitals. For many parents, however, this is enormously disturbing, and they will go to great lengths to stop any such genital exploration. I firmly believe that this kind of reaction sets the stage for sexual difficulties later in life. The parents have introduced and reinforced the idea that touching genitals and the feelings associated with that elicits disapproval from the most important people in their lives.

In response to your last question, you can't pinpoint one moment when children become sexual persons. Certainly with the onset of puberty—ages 10 to 11 in girls, 12 to 13 in boys—young people begin to have explicit sexual feelings along with the surge in hormones. As teenagers, they may have experienced physical sensations earlier, but these feelings are intimately tied to their increased awareness and knowledge.

> **When my husband and I go on vacation, we often have our 18-month-old son sleep in the same bedroom with us. I am uncomfortable having sex when he's there, even if he is asleep. My husband thinks I'm being ridiculous. What do you think?**

Your concerns are valid; it's one thing to be open with your children about sex, providing them with information and helping them feel comfortable with their bodies. It's quite another matter to let them witness an act that they may find frightening and confusing. Many people make a variety of noises during sex that children might interpret as symptoms of pain or distress. And once involved in lovemaking, few couples are likely to notice if their child has awakened and is listening or watching.

With discretion, however, it is possible for you and your husband to make love in this situation. Having sex quietly and under the covers is okay if your son is asleep and you are comfortable doing it. Anything less discreet risks waking him up and exposing him to something potentially upsetting.

> **I've got three children: a boy and two girls, ages 2, 4, and 7, respectively. I usually let them all bathe together because they seem to have fun and it's easier for me. Lately, the 7-year-old has started asking to shower on her own. I'm not sure how to respond.**

There really aren't any hard-and-fast rules regarding children bathing together. In my opinion, it's harmless and often presents interesting opportunities for you and your children to talk about bodies and differences between girls and boys in a setting that is comfortable and fun. It also provides an opportunity to begin talking about respect for people's physical boundaries and can be a forerunner to teaching about the need and right to some privacy.

As far as your older daughter is concerned, however, she's growing up, and she's indicated that she's no longer comfortable with group bathing. You should honor her needs and wishes. You can help her put her feelings into words by telling her that, now that she's older, she wants more privacy. Explain to her and your other children that the desire for privacy is healthy and should be respected. It might be a good time to talk about learning to knock on a closed door before entering.

> **Should parents walk around in their underwear in front of their kids?**

The question of modesty and nudity is a very personal one. Some people see the human body as an object of beauty to be displayed and admired, and nudity is acceptable to them. Others consider the body to be a private matter.

Here are some of my guidelines when it comes to nudity: Same-sex nudity between parent and child can be fine, providing a way for kids to notice things about their own bodies and a safe opportunity for them to express curiosity. With sons and mothers or fathers and daughters, I think there should be a thoughtful consideration of boundaries. I don't think that sons should bathe with their mothers after the age of 2, and likewise, fathers need to be discreet with their daughters. I do not mean to be dogmatic and judgmental, and there are many situations where the level of comfort and openness of parents may override these guidelines.

For some families, walking around in underwear may be fine because it feels totally natural. If, however, someone is uncomfortable with it (whether parent or child), those feelings need to be discussed and respected.

Also, keep in mind that when kids become teenagers, they require more privacy when it comes to their bodies. Parents need to be especially understanding of the heightened sensitivity of teens while going through puberty and be respectful and not demeaning.

> I recently walked in on my 5-year-old son "playing doctor" with his 4-year-old cousin. She was lying on the floor with her clothes off. I tried to be cool and said that she ought to get dressed and I would give them both a snack. What should I have done?

Remember, there is rarely an absolute "right" solution. As parents, we are often confronted with situations for which we've had no preparation. We do our best, and we improvise. In the incident you mention, it sounds as if your son and niece were expressing a normal, healthy curiosity.

Noticing bodily differences is particularly intriguing for children. I remember the story of the little girl who saw her baby brother in the bathtub for first time and said to her mother, "Thank goodness he doesn't have that on his face!"

I think you handled the situation well; you didn't get angry or give the kids the impression that they were doing something bad. I would suggest, however, that you have a follow-up discussion with your son. Ask him what he and his cousin were doing, and what he thinks about the ways their bodies are different from each other. You could use the opportunity to educate him about the male and female bodies. It's better that you do the educating, rather than television shows, magazines, and movies. The incident may have been disturbing to you initially, but it's a wonderful opportunity for you and your spouse to begin talking to your child about bodies and boundaries.

> My 12-year-old daughter was running on the track at school. As she ran past a group of boys, one reached out and pinched her rear end. She was terribly upset and wondered what she did to deserve this. Her coach told her that it was just a joke and to forget it, but I cannot forget how upset she was when she came home. What would you do?

You know it is easy to slough this off and simply say, "Big deal, boys will be boys!" This happens every day in schools across the country, but I believe that it promotes actions that demean girls and leads to the acceptance of behavior we now call harassment. It should *not* be ignored because it makes those who experience it feel shame, embarrassment, and sometimes responsibility.

Adults like that coach fail our children by not being clear that such behavior crosses acceptable boundaries. As a parent, you should speak to the teachers and guidance counselors and insist that they educate your daughter's peers by giving this activity a name—sexual harassment. Girls need to be able to speak out on the topic, and boys need to understand that they do not have the right to behave this way.

Your daughter should get an apology from the boy—and the coach. She is entitled to the chance to state clearly and publicly that she does not want boys touching her body, and they need to hear that they have hurt her feelings.

Teens and Sex

Adolescence is a challenge to the most hardy parents. The range of possible crises adolescents can confront one with boggles the mind. Today's teens are having sex earlier and with more partners. A fact paper from the Center for Population (1994) reports the following:

* Approximately 40% of both boys and girls between the ages of 15 and 19 years used ineffective or no contraception at first intercourse.
* Planned initiation of intercourse among teenagers is rare. Only 17% of girls and 25% of boys reported planning their first intercourse.
* As of September 1992, 10,182 cases of acquired immunodeficiency syndrome (AIDS) among young people (ages 13–24 years) had been reported to the Centers for Disease Control and Prevention (CDC). In addition, nearly 20% of persons with AIDS are 20–29 years old. Given the average 10-year latency period between human immunodeficiency virus (HIV) infection and onset of AIDS symptoms, many of these individuals were infected with AIDS during their teenage years.

When it comes to sex, parents too often equate discussions and knowledge about sexuality with encouraging their children to have intercourse. I like to think of it as providing children with the information they need to begin to think through for themselves what sexuality is about and to begin to think about what a shared relationship is about.

I'm confused about what exactly happens to girls and boys during puberty.

Puberty is the stage of adolescent development associated with the onset of sexual development and maturity. The sex hormones (testosterone for boys, estrogen and progesterone for girls) are produced by the body in increasing amounts. This increase is associated with a physical growth spurt, voice changes, development of breasts, enlargement of penis and testicles, and growth of pubic hair. Boys produce sperm and semen and may have nocturnal ejaculations called "wet dreams"; girls begin to menstruate. The changes during this period are as great as the changes in the first 2 years of life. There is a growth surge and the adolescent's body seems to change almost daily; you will often notice adolescents' clumsiness, caused by their need to learn their new spatial relationships. The surge in sex hormones also leads to powerful sexual feelings; boys will have spontaneous erections many times a day, and girls will feel the tingling sensations associated with sexual arousal. The emotional ups and downs are a challenge at this time to both adolescents and their parents!

> **I was startled to hear that at least 30% of all 15-year-olds have had intercourse. Would you comment on that?**

I don't know how to say it forcefully enough: Most teens are simply not ready emotionally to have sexual intercourse, and we need to provide them with good reasons why it makes sense for them to wait.

This is an area where I think many parents let their kids down by not providing useful guidelines. Telling them to "just say no" is not adequate or believable advice. By the time parents are struggling with the idea that their teen may be having sex, it's too late. Both Mom and Dad need to convey a consistent set of values by sharing their attitudes about sexuality early on.

Suzi Landolphi covers this issue warmly and directly in her book *Hot, Sexy, and Safer* (see the appendix ["Information Resources"] at the end of this book). In it, she focuses on how parents can help their kids develop healthy self-esteem, provide them with reliable information and guidance, and be available for open, honest discussions. I would encourage parents to read this book; I wish it had been available when I was a teenager.

> My 15-year-old brother seems sex-hungry. He had sex with a girl for the first time when he was 13. Since then, he's dated many girls—sometimes two different ones in a week— and has slept with many of them. I'm 17 and only recently started wanting to have a girlfriend. Is he oversexed or am I missing something?

Frankly, I think that he is the one missing something. He may brag about his accomplishments and ridicule you, but I think he is being ruled by his hormones, not his brain. I do believe, however, that we grown-ups give confusing and contradictory messages when it comes to teens and sex. The current climate of explicit television shows and movies promotes a precocious "learned" sexuality. What's more, sex in advertising conveys powerful messages aimed at the young. While parents are trying to encourage caution and restraint, kids are being bombarded with signals that say sex is power, sex is cool, sex is *now*.

Parents can provide some guidance and guidelines that value relationships over sex. When a teen behaves in a sexually precocious way, the sex usually fills the need for something else that is missing. For boys, being sexual and "scoring" are equated with being cool and strong. Again, I think that we all bear some responsibility for perpetuating this myth. For girls, sexual compliance may be a way of feeling needed, feeling popular, or feeling more powerful.

A more complicated explanation may also relate to some feelings that the parents may not have worked out satisfactorily for themselves. They may inadvertently encourage the children to behave in a way that fulfills their own unrecognized conflicts. A man who feels sexually threatened may not be aware that he is encouraging his son's sexual behavior as a way to feel better himself. I have seen women who viewed sex as a way of enhancing their self-esteem indirectly encourage their daughters to enter prematurely into sexual relationships.

I recently walked into my 12-year-old son's bedroom and found him masturbating with another boy. I was mortified, and so were they. I turned around immediately and left. I didn't bring it up later and neither did he. What should I do now?

Let me reassure you that what you describe is common, normal behavior. When boys first go through puberty and begin to masturbate, they sometimes do it with friends. This is a process of discovery and developing awareness, and they find comfort in doing it with a friend. You can use this situation to begin or continue discussions about sexual feelings. (Using a spontaneous event as a springboard for discussion usually works much better than the formal "let's sit down and have a talk" approach.)

You both know what you have seen, and by not talking, you send the subtle message that it is too terrible to be discussed. Apologize for your intrusion and acknowledge that you were embarrassed, as was he. You might agree that everyone in the family should knock before opening a closed bedroom door. Additionally, I would hope that you and your husband might think about how to continue a dialogue. All too often, mothers are left to handle these situations, and it is a loss for both sons and fathers that the male parent does not take a more active role. Most men I have spoken to report that the only conversation they had with their fathers about sex had to do with the need to "be careful" and little else.

How common is masturbation among teenagers?

Studies have shown that most teenage boys and many teenage girls masturbate. Certainly it is the most prevalent form of sexual activity in adolescence, with some kids masturbating almost every day and other kids barely at all. If it is viewed as an activity that is part of becoming a sexual adult and a way of discovering one's sexual feelings and deriving pleasure from one's body, it can be an advantage on the way to adult sexual relationships. Regrettably, for many it is still associated with feelings of shame and embarrassment.

Should parents encourage their kids to masturbate?

Parents should neither encourage nor discourage masturbation. Conveying comfort and acceptance of one's sexual feelings can be one of the greatest gifts a parent can give. By the time kids are 9 or 10, it's best to have talked to them about the changes their bodies will be going through and to have explained that they will be aware of a new set of "sexual" feelings as their bodies grow and mature. The idea is to present sex as a normal part of life without telling children to act on it before they have any inclination. You might get an age-appropriate book to help break the ice. Despite the talk about masturbation being okay, many people still feel conflicted about either doing it or recognizing that their children do it. There is the story of the 12-year-old boy who was found masturbating by a parent. "Don't do that—you'll go blind!" said the parent. "Can I do it until I need glasses?" asked the boy.

I know that my 16-year-old son is sexually active, and I don't approve. I feel that my saying anything is pointless because I cannot control his activities.

You probably are right that you cannot stop him from engaging in sex. A more productive thing for you to do at this point is to identify your concerns about his activities, such as health and safety issues and contraception. You need to think through your ideas about sexuality for teens by asking yourself these questions:

* What was my experience as a teen?
* What did I want to know?
* What did I want help understanding?
* What experiences were good? bad?
* What do I think about teen sexuality now?
* What values do I want to convey?

Once you have done that—and I would suggest your husband be a part of this—think about when the two of you could have a discussion with your son. It may break the ice to start off with something like, "We want to talk with you about sex—we both feel nervous about doing this and it will probably be uncomfortable for you and for us—but let's forge ahead and see what we can do." Remember, you have not had experience or training with this; it is new and uncomfortable, and the only way to get better at it is to practice. He may not thank you for the input, but he will know from your words that you care deeply about his physical and psychological health.

> Is fear of AIDS changing the way teens behave? Are their practices different? Their attitudes? As a parent of three teens, I'm hoping that AIDS awareness educational campaigns have gotten the message across better than I could.

My informal surveys of medical students give anecdotal evidence that abstinence is on the rise. Other data show that after more than a decade of rapid increases in the number of teens having sexual intercourse, the increase is slowing. Still, many teens are having sex, and there's solid evidence that many do not use condoms. Recently, I was startled to find that in one medical school first-year class, 25% (both men and women) said that they had engaged in risky sex within the past year! A more educated, highly motivated, goal-directed group would be hard to find. Clearly, it is not just kids who think AIDS and pregnancy cannot happen to them. Because AIDS is an incurable illness, parents, doctors, and educators are faced with a very important challenge: How do we talk to kids about this in a believable, convincing way? The key is to be direct, open, and honest. Give children solid information without using fear tactics. You might start with a discussion of other risky behaviors: smoking cigarettes, driving without a seat belt, riding a motorcycle without a helmet, walking in an unsafe area late at night. Then discuss the dangers of unprotected and premature sex.

Kids must have reliable, current information. So shed whatever notion you have about what children should or shouldn't know, and be prepared to tackle tough issues. If you need to educate yourself first, do. No one can afford to let children they are responsible for rely on myths and misinformation spread through the grapevine. Schools and some nonprofit organizations are becoming more creative in the ways they handle issues around safety, AIDS awareness, and choices to delay sexual activity. Planned Parenthood has an excellent program that focuses on assessing risk and finding ways to choose abstinence. What is impressive about this program is that it involves young "trainers" who are seen as more genuine and believable than old folks over 30!

> **My son is 15 and has expressed no interest at all in girls. I think he may be homosexual. What should I do?**

Not having dated girls by age 15 is *not* a sign of latent homosexuality. It's not unusual for boys to stay in their shell with the opposite sex until college or even later. Similarly, some men come to realize that they are homosexual later in life, after having been intimate with one or more women. There also are, of course, kids who know that they are "different" very early on and who carry that knowledge as a burden for years without talking to either a parent or another helping adult.

As a parent, you may have several reasons, perhaps ones that you can't quite put into words, for wondering whether your son is gay. The only way to find out is to maintain open and supportive communication with him. If he is gay, and if he recognizes that about himself, in time he will tell you.

If your family has a history of openness, you could say, "Look, I'm wondering if you have questions about your sexual orientation. Is that something you want to talk about?" For many parents, this might be extremely difficult. To some degree, I think it is probably best left to the teen to bring it up. However, this will not happen if there are powerful cues in the family that homosexuality is deviant, bad, and not to be tolerated. Certainly, all parents should be prepared to share their attitudes about same-sex relationships if a child brings up the subject.

If your child confides to you that he is gay, ask why he thinks so. It is quite common for kids to experiment sexually with friends of the same gender. It's not surprising that they may be more comfortable touching the type of body that they know. Often, this kind of interest is just a passing phase. The point is not to label your child's behavior.

It's crucial that parents not respond to a child's concern about homosexuality by asking, "What did I do wrong?" That only makes kids feel guilty when what they are seeking is reassurance and love.

Why do some children grow up to be gay?

The question of what causes a child to become a lesbian or homosexual adult is very controversial. The basic answer is that we don't know. Current theory is that it has more to do with genetics and biology than was previously thought. Many of the hypotheses people used to come up with—for example, that homosexual males have domineering mothers and passive fathers—have been discredited. We all know people who had parents like that who grew up to be heterosexual.

One other thing: Generally speaking, a person favors either a heterosexual or homosexual orientation throughout his or her life. But there are many instances where someone who consistently had same-sex partners met and fell in love with an opposite-sex partner and vice versa. It is clear that sexual orientation is a very complicated matter.

C*hapter 10*

Childhood Sexual Abuse

*F*reud was onto something in Vienna, the full impact of which was not clear to him. He was impressed with the number of women who told him that as children they had had some form of sexual experience with a parent or other adult. This led him initially to develop a theory to explain "hysteria"—a phenomenon in which people developed what seemed to be neurological symptoms without demonstrable disease.

He was disturbed, however, by the fact that he knew many of the parents of his patients, and he could not believe that the sexual encounters described had really occurred. This led him to conclude that his theory must be wrong, and to develop an alternative explanation for his patients' symptoms. He proposed that, rather than having actually experienced such encounters, his patients possessed unconscious desires and longings to be sexual with parents or other adults, and that the guilt around these thoughts caused their symptoms. Although this theory seems far-fetched today, one has to keep in mind that this was the late 1890s in Vienna, when the Victorian influence on repressing sexual urges was in full swing.

I remember my own experiences when patients would tell me

about awful things that had happened to them as children. I found it hard to believe them for a few reasons. The first had to do with my limited "worldly experience"; I simply could not imagine that degree of assault against a child. The second and more complicated reason was the apparent absence of feeling while these people related hideous experiences. They appeared calm and removed, as if they were discussing the weather, and this lent an air of unreality to what I was hearing.

We have come a long way in our understanding. We know that the incidence of childhood sexual abuse in both girls and boys is appallingly high (15%–25%), and this is across socioeconomic lines. We have come to understand that children protect themselves against this kind of assault by mentally removing or "dissociating" themselves from their bodies.

Many adults who were abused as children have learned very effectively to shut off the feelings (and in many instances the memories) associated with this abuse. While shutting off feelings served a purpose in childhood, it becomes a huge hindrance for the adults; people who have suffered childhood sexual abuse are more likely as adults to land in exploitative relationships (sexually, physically, or emotionally). The warning signals that might indicate to them that they are in some form of danger don't get through because when they were children they learned to tune out and shut down in these situations, and this mechanism continues to operate.

Topics covered in this chapter include the following:

* Should I tell my partner about childhood sexual abuse?
* My husband was sexually abused
* Long-term effects of sexual abuse in childhood
* Treatment for adult survivors of childhood sexual abuse
* Treatment outcome

I was sexually abused as a child by my father beginning at 8 and lasting until I was 11. I now live with a man I really care

for and am afraid to tell him about the abuse. I worry it will change his feelings toward me. But I also feel I should be honest. What would you do?

First let me say how sorry I am that you had to endure this assault. You are not alone. Because of the shame surrounding sexual abuse, researchers do not know for certain how many people are abused, but some guess the number is as high as one in six people.

It is understandably difficult to tell someone close to you about such a trauma. One of the cruelest consequences in these cases is that victims are robbed of the ability to trust. Abused children feel as if they have no one to protect them and no one with whom they can share their secret. As adults, they struggle with opening up to their partners and worry that they will not be believed, or worse, that they will be rejected.

If your relationship is based on caring and reciprocity, you may find it a relief to talk with your boyfriend. If he is compassionate, he is likely to validate your feelings and become an even greater source of support in your life. If you sometimes shy away from sex, he should understand why and help you work through your fears rather than berate you.

There is a chance he may retreat; men sometimes feel threatened when hearing about earlier abuse because initially they focus on the "sexual" and don't see the violence and danger. I have seen situations in which partner's reactions are insensitive, and I think that this is another instance where a professional can help explain what has happened and help the couple get the understanding and support they need.

I suggest that you look into a support group for survivors of sexual abuse. You may find it easier to open up with others who have had similar experiences, and hearing how others have healed can give you some hope.

My husband and I have been happily married for 15 years. Over the past few months, he has begun to have recollections of being sexually abused repeatedly by an uncle from the ages of 9 to 15. He has had terrible nightmares and finds it very hard to make love. What would you advise?

The changes in your husband's behavior will be easier to understand if you realize the devastation that childhood sexual abuse can bring to a child's psyche. Perpetrators can be either adults or other children. Most commonly they are relatives, as in your husband's case—even parents. The abuse can range from inappropriate fondling to forcing children to engage in oral sex or intercourse.

The shame and guilt that children feel often keeps them from telling an adult—and when they do, their accounts often are not believed. Sexual abuse commonly leaves children with no place to turn. This type of attack is so painful and overwhelming, many children deal with it by separating their mind from their body into something known as a *dissociative state*. This protects them, even as terrible things are happening to their bodies.

Although dissociation provides some protection at the moment the abuse is occurring, it can create a pattern that leaves the victim emotionally numb. That numbness carries into adult life, and unless the individual is aware of this, the consequences may be severe.

A problem in treating sexually abused people is that they often have little or no conscious recall of what happened. As children, they were so helpless that they totally blocked out the trauma. Denial helps them survive but costs them dearly later. When they reach adulthood, they may suddenly experience flashbacks—body sensations similar to what they felt during abuse. One woman described a recurrent choking sensation. After she saw a television program on sexual abuse, memories of having to perform oral sex on her father came flooding back. Others report flashbacks being set off by daily stress or anxiety.

In recent years, controversy has erupted over experiences such as your husband's, in which a person with no previous memory of abuse and who has enjoyed healthy adult sexual relationships suddenly experiences anxiety, nightmares, physical symptoms, and

flashbacks. Recently, there have been legal challenges to these recollections, leading to the concept of the "false memory syndrome."
I believe that there may be some instances in which therapists are
overzealous in their attempts to elicit memories of childhood abuse,
but in other cases, the diagnosis of false memory syndrome is, I
believe, a dangerous reaction to the discomfort people feel about
admitting that these events do occur.

Professional treatment is essential. It usually is the only way
for survivors to understand what has happened and shed their awful
feelings. For now, be supportive of your husband, and encourage
him to get help. His aversion to making love may increase initially,
but with support and guidance, he should be able to reclaim his
sexual feelings. Keep in mind that for victims of abuse, the connection between sexual feelings and danger is very strong. To be
sexual is to open themselves to those very scary feelings. It's crucial
for victims to regain a sense of being able to control what happens
to them; this means that you have to be patient and not insist that
your husband resume sex prematurely. Feeling safe is the forerunner of being sexual.

By gently reestablishing a sexual relationship, your husband
will learn what sexual activities stir bad memories. Recognizing that
he is with someone who is caring and responsive will help modify
his responses. Although at times it may be very difficult, try to
avoid anger. Inevitably the partners of victims of abuse feel rejected
themselves, but anger will result in your husband feeling as he did
as a child.

What long-lasting effects do victims of childhood sexual abuse experience?

First of all, a number of factors can influence the severity of these
effects:

* The age at which the abuse first occurred. Generally, the earlier the abuse, the worse the consequences.
* The degree of abuse and the type of force used.

* The threat of repercussions. Children who are told they will be killed if they tell anyone, or that God will punish them, experience deep-seated fears well into adulthood.
* Who the abuser was. When it is a parent, the effects are particularly devastating because of the total breakdown of the child's safety net.
* How parents react when they find out about the abuse. If an adult supports and reassures the child by sending him or her to counseling, the effects will be minimized because the child will regain some sense of protection.

Men and women who underwent such abuse typically have terrible self-image problems. There are exceptions, of course, but most feel some guilt or shame about what was done to them. They may go through periods of sexual promiscuity, having many sexual partners yet deriving no pleasure from the encounters. Often they enter relationships and end them without knowing why. They don't understand that the experience of being close with someone stirs up feelings of danger and that running away from intimacy is a self-protective response.

This emotional vulnerability makes survivors of childhood sexual abuse more likely to get into dangerous sexual situations. The numbing mechanism they used as children blocks their recognition of danger signals. Because self-esteem is such a pivotal issue in sexuality, victims of abuse typically have problems with desire, arousal, giving and receiving pleasure, and achieving orgasm. After sex, they may become terribly, inexplicably sad.

How do you treat an adult who was sexually abused as a child?

Talking therapy is usually a central part of people's recovery. Having a relationship with an adult with whom the experiences can be shared and with whom they can feel safe is very helpful. Medication is sometimes used, along with behavioral therapy. Because every person is different, the approach has to be individual, and the time for successful treatment can vary considerably, from a few months to several years. The healing process—feeling safe in a relationship and believing that they deserve to be loved and treated well—is a slow one.

Often a patient seeks help because he or she is unable to engage in or enjoy intercourse or other types of physical intimacy. It's important to know that that's okay. Part of the process of healing is reclaiming control of one's body. Once therapy has begun and the individual begins to feel safer emotionally, I generally suggest a series of structured sexual exercises that limit the range of activity. This allows the patient to pinpoint what makes him or her uncomfortable and to express that to the partner—something that was never possible as a child.

Having an understanding partner is critical. Often, the victim is uncomfortable during lovemaking but feels guilty saying so because of the partner's frustration. It is essential that the victim know it is okay to say, "No. I don't want to do that." When treating the couple, I always talk with the partner to help him or her know what's going on.

By slowly recalling the early events, the patient can learn to cast off much of the trauma and commit to a relationship in which he or she is valued, loved, and treated well. Supervised mediation with the abuser—where the victim works with the perpetrator face-to-face—may be useful in some situations. However, it is not essential, and it is a mistake to push this on someone who does not wish to do it.

Does treatment always work with victims of childhood sexual abuse?

Regrettably, no. Sometimes the abuse has left such deep marks on a person's psyche that the pain can only be controlled, not cured. Other times, a therapist might suspect abuse as the root of a serious sexual or psychological problem and may even raise the question. Unless the individual can recall an incident, there is no way to uncover what happened.

In my own practice, I once treated a couple for whom sex therapy only made matters worse. Although they had been together about 14 years, the wife could not bear being touched by her husband. She loved him and he loved her, and in all other realms their relationship was good, but touching elicited a visceral reaction that she could not control. I learned that her mother had been very quiet, somewhat mousy, and terrified of her father. He was a burly man who had a serious alcohol problem that resulted in frequent enraged outbursts.

I suggested that the couple try the sensate focus exercises that Masters and Johnson had developed (see pages 101–102). There is nothing magical or mysterious about these—they are simply designed to help people focus attention on the physical sensations and help shift the emphasis away from performance to pleasure. I try to present them in a loose way: take turns in exploring touch; use a combination of kissing, massage, and stroking; switch roles, with one giving and the other receiving, and then alternate roles; and finally, leave breasts and genitals off limits. This final instruction often surprises people. The reason for the prohibition is that couples often focus on the genital performance so much that sexual experience in shared touch is missing.

This couple did not do well with the exercises. The wife talked about feeling enraged and angry, though she could not understand why. We proceeded with this for a few weeks; I tried to have her control what was happening, and there was some improvement. The next phase involved some genital caressing. When the couple came to their session, the wife talked about feeling in a rage, wanting to attack her husband's penis as if she were wringing out a dishrag, and having dreams that her teeth and gums were falling out. I became concerned with her reactions and felt that the sex therapy was becoming harmful. I believed that there was some awful experience that she could not yet remember (my hunch was that her alcoholic father had sexually abused her) and that the therapy, with its explicit instructions to have genital and body caressing, was replicating something that was truly disturbing. I interrupted the couple's therapy and urged her to seek out individual counseling.

I believe there has been a backlash against victims of sexual abuse in the form of the viewpoint that the memories are false. Regrettably, there are therapists who may have been overzealous in trying to elicit memories, and there are many publicized accounts of parents or relatives being falsely accused. The important issue is this: Sexual abuse of children is a common and terrible problem, and as a society we have to face it.

In some situations, one parent *was* a victim of sexual abuse, and although that parent's own children were not abused, somehow the children have picked up the parent's sense of fearfulness and lack of safety. People who have grown up in such an environment may appear to therapists to be victims of abuse, but I would describe them more as "vicarious victims." The legacies of their parents' abuse cause them emotional difficulties that require treatment.

Chapter 11

Surgery and Illness

The older people get, the more likely they are to have a serious medical condition that requires medication or surgery. Recovery in many situations may not be complete, and the individual has to deal with impaired functioning of varying degrees. Too often, people are dealt with as if the illness had no bearing on other aspects of their lives and psyches. Usually, health care providers pay no attention to their patients' sexual well-being. People notice this silence, and it discourages many from broaching the topic with their physicians. Medicines have side effects, illnesses may result in lowered sexual desire, and surgeries may result in major changes in body image.

Topics covered in this chapter include the following:

* Hysterectomy and changes in sexual feelings
* Resuming sex after a heart attack
* Sex problems after mastectomy for breast cancer
* Effects of prostate surgery on sex
* Diminished sexual interest after colon surgery
* Chronic illness and sexual functioning
* Antidepressants and sex

*H*ysterectomy

My doctor has recommended that I have a hysterectomy. But I am only 35 and worried about how this operation will affect my sex drive. What kind of changes can I expect?

Your question is extremely important, and I hope it encourages all readers to educate themselves whenever a doctor suggests a medical or surgical technique. The more you know about what is involved in the surgery, the better you'll adjust. Ask your doctor questions; talk to people who have had the operation; and if you have nagging doubts, consider a second opinion before proceeding. In the past decade, a wider array of alternatives has allowed many women to choose between hysterectomy and nonsurgical options.

If you choose hysterectomy, you'll have lots of company. By age 60, one of three women in the United States has had a hysterectomy. A brief anatomical review will help illustrate some of what happens after the procedure: Your uterus is a pear-shaped organ with a fallopian tube on each side. Next to each fallopian tube is an ovary that produces the hormone estrogen and stores eggs. At the bottom of the uterus is the cervix, a ring of tissue with a very small opening through which the menstrual blood flows and sperm enter from the vagina.

All hysterectomies end menstruation and the ability to get pregnant. There are different ways of doing a hysterectomy. One approach is to remove the uterus through the vagina, which may shorten recovery time after the operation. It may be necessary to perform the surgery by making an incision in the abdominal wall, which will result in a longer recovery. There are reasons for the different approaches, which your gynecologist will discuss. In some instances, only the uterus is removed. If the ovaries are removed along with the uterus, the body's main source of female hormones is taken away, and surgical "menopause" results. Hormone replacement therapy is often recommended, especially for younger women.

After surgery, the vaginal canal may shorten because of loss of tissue, though with time it will stretch out again. If the cervix is removed, you will no longer feel the pressure of the penis pushing on it during intercourse, which some women enjoy. Be aware that after your uterus is removed, you will no longer feel its contractions during orgasm. You still will have orgasms, but they will feel different.

It usually takes 4 to 6 weeks to recover from the surgery. Some women feel diminished sexual interest much longer, caused by either hormonal changes or a mourning of the loss of the uterus and fertility. Still other women find that hysterectomy provides an enhanced sense of well-being. Knowing what to expect helps the adjustment, and sex can once again become an enjoyable, fulfilling experience.

*H*eart Attack

> I'm 53, and about a year ago I had a heart attack. I'm fully recovered and exercise regularly, which my doctor said was okay. But my wife and I have been too embarrassed to ask if we can resume sex, too.

I'll bet your doctor never raised the subject, either! So many people worry after a heart attack that they will precipitate another by having sex. Sex can be a great source of life-affirming comfort and pleasure, however. It should not be avoided; you need to discuss your concerns openly with your cardiologist.

The usual guidelines about exercise after a heart attack relate to whether the patient gets short of breath or develops chest pain. Most often, people are placed on an exercise regimen, followed by periodic stress tests (more strenuous than most sex!). Chances are you can start making love again if you are exercising. But, as I said before, talk with your doctor first. If your doctor is reluctant or uncomfortable about giving you an answer, ask if he or she knows someone who has the information that you are seeking. I know this may feel awkward, but there is much information that can be help-ful, and you need access to it.

Breast Cancer

> **Several years ago, I was diagnosed with breast cancer. I had one breast removed. Now I'm fine, but sex with my husband isn't the same. It seems as if we're both inhibited. What's going on?**

The removal of a breast because of cancer is a trauma for everyone involved. Both the woman's and her partner's lives are turned up-side down, and the mastectomy is a constant reminder that life has forever changed. This is a time of enormous stress, and couples may be frightened to discuss their concerns and worries openly with each other. Too often, women feel shame about the change in their bodies, and husbands feel too frightened to be supportive. The worry about recurrence, the effect of the radiation or chemo-therapy treatments, and the many decisions to be made overload the couple. The woman may be shy about her body, her partner may avoid looking at it, and the mastectomy may become a symbol of all the emotions and fears it holds hostage.

In therapy, I try to guide people to focus on their priorities. Preserving life rather than emphasizing cosmetics should be the main goal. Providing support and comfort for one another is really what makes dealing with cancer manageable.

> **How do you treat people who have sexual problems after mastectomy?**

When a couple comes to me, they usually are in a state of shock. They've been through a nightmare of treatment decisions, surgery, and recovery. They feel confused and worried about the future. Each is trying to deal with his or her own reactions and trying to offer support to the other. They often have children about whom they are also concerned. Generally, if sex was good before the surgery, it will be easier for the couple to adapt and to resume sexual relations. Therapy is aimed at getting the wife to talk about her concerns and reactions to the changes in her body. The husband must think about his reactions, too, and share them with his wife.

Couples need to know that it is all right to feel squeamish about the scar. I encourage them to resume touching each other as soon as possible and remind them to focus on their relationship and their feelings for each other. Restoring their sexual relationship provides a couple with comfort and reassurance that helps them resume their lives.

*P*rostate Surgery

I'm 65 and was recently told by my urologist that I need prostate surgery. Is that going to affect my sex life?

As men get older, the prostate gland that surrounds the urethra (the passage from the bladder out through the penis) usually becomes enlarged, a condition called benign prostatic hypertrophy (BPH). BPH does not always produce symptoms. However, if it makes urinating difficult, it requires treatment, which may involve surgery. There are two basic types of prostate surgery:

* *Transurethral resection (TUR)* is performed through the penis. Erectile functioning is usually not impaired. There may be "retrograde ejaculation," where the semen goes into the bladder instead of out through the penis.
* *Suprapubic prostatectomy* involves more extensive surgery that may result in some inadvertent damages to the nerves in the area, causing impotence. Orgasm is usually fine (if no nerves have been damaged), though there is no ejaculate, which is often viewed as a loss.

It is important to discuss the surgical options and the reasons your urologist recommends a particular one. You may need a biopsy so that a piece of the prostate tissue can be examined under a microscope. If there is evidence of cancer, many urologists recommend radiation therapy or a combination of surgery and radiation.

Most men have considerable psychological anxiety associated with any surgery close to the penis, and this worry may result in erectile difficulties not related to physical damage from the surgery. The more you and your wife know about what to expect, the better prepared you will be. Many urology practices have a team approach, with trained counselors who can provide information and reassurance about sexual functioning.

Colon Surgery

I have been happily married to a wonderful man for over 30 years. We have been close and have always enjoyed sex. However, he had surgery for colon cancer about a year ago that resulted in a colostomy. Since that time, he's hardly interested in sex at all. I know that the surgery took a toll on him, and I don't want to add to that by letting him know my own frustration. What would you advise?

It is sad when the pain and suffering of a chronic illness are made worse by affecting a couple's sexual relationship. Counseling can make a big difference; your husband and you could use help in putting the illness and surgery into perspective and talking about what it means to him. The sense of shame around the changes in the body often results in feeling unattractive and believing that the spouse is disgusted and turned off. Invariably, people feel depressed, and this too needs treatment. The counselor can help both of you tap into the resources of the relationship and provide mutual support. If sex was a source of enjoyment and comfort before the surgery, it is important to have that outlet available.

Chronic Illness and Sexual Functioning

Chronic physical illnesses that can disturb a couple's sexual patterns include heart disease and heart attack, stroke, cancer, diabetes, severe arthritis, and neurological disorders such as multiple sclerosis. The medications used to treat these illnesses also may cause serious sexual difficulties. The emotional effects of chronic ill health on an individual are profound, and unfortunately often ignored by physicians. For example:

* Illness creates a heightened sense of vulnerability. The patient can no longer take health for granted, and this can shake confidence regarding all things having to do with the body.
* Self-esteem may suffer. The patient may be sensitive about the changes in the body and may feel defective and scarred and be ashamed to be seen naked.
* Anxieties about general health, treatment, and the financial impact of illness may become overwhelming.
* The illness may leave the patient depressed, which in turn depresses sexual functioning and desire.
* Both partners may worry that the exertion of sex is harmful.
* Given the woeful lack of information about sex, if genital intercourse is not an option, the couple may not know any other behaviors that can bring them sexual satisfaction.

If your physician does not address the following issues, bring them up yourself:

* What effects will this condition or procedure have on my sexual functioning?
* Do these medications impair sexual functioning?
* Can you suggest anything I/we can read to get more information?
* Can you refer my spouse and me to someone who can help us confront some of the changes we're facing?

Depression

Serious depression affects more than 11 million adults every year, but only one-third of them seek treatment. There are several types of depressive illness, any one of which can have a dramatic and debilitating effect on a person's sex life.

When you describe someone as "depressed," the common assumption is that you are talking about someone with a serious mental disturbance who can't work or function. In reality, clinical depression can provoke a wide range of responses:

* Sadness, irritability, guilt, or hopelessness
* Loss of interest or pleasure in activities once enjoyed
* Change in weight, appetite, or sleep patterns
* Inability to concentrate, remember things, or make decisions
* Little interest in or pleasure from sex
* Fatigue or loss of energy
* Restlessness or decreased activity
* Complaints of physical aches and pains for which no medical explanation can be found
* Thoughts of death or suicide

Over the years, I have treated many couples in which one partner was depressed. Each person and situation is different, but in every case, when one person was depressed, the whole family was affected. Ideally, the partner will be patient, understanding, and will provide assistance and encouragement. But this can be difficult, especially when family members feel a loss because the depressed person is less available emotionally, or are saddened by the pain that the depressed person so obviously feels.

Compounding the difficulties is that, almost inevitably, depression affects a couple's sexual relationship. The most common complaint is a lack of desire—simply not feeling in the mood. If the couple does have sex, it usually is devoid of excitement and joy.

Drug Treatment for Depression

Drugs used to treat depression—*antidepressants*—typically take effect slowly. It may be 4 weeks or longer before the individual feels better. If sex has previously been enjoyable and satisfying, the improved mood will be reflected in better sex. If the sexual relationship had difficulties before the depression, the couple is now in a position to tackle that problem directly. One complicating factor is that in some instances, the antidepressant adversely affects sexual functioning (see question below). It is not possible to predict who will be affected, and in some instances the treatment of the depression is the overriding concern. Antidepressant drugs can be grouped into several categories, including the following:

* **Paxil, Prozac, Zoloft, and Effexor**—These selective serotonin reuptake inhibitors (SSRIs) are among the newly developed antidepressants that work by affecting the brain's natural chemical messengers. Because their action is so specifically targeted, they have fewer side effects than other antidepressants. For this reason, they have become widely prescribed. Still, reactions to these drugs vary from person to person.
* **Nardil, Parnate**—These drugs, known as monoamine oxidase inhibitors (MAOIs), have been used extensively in Europe for many years. In the United States, psychiatrists have been reluctant to prescribe them because a serious rise in blood pressure is a possible side effect. When prescribed by an experienced practitioner, however, and given to patients with very specific diet instructions, they can be extremely effective.
* **Elavil, Norpramin, Tofranil, and others**—Although very effective, commonly used, and well tested, the tricyclic antidepressants (TCAs) are associated with many side effects, including blurred vision, blood pressure difficulties, constipation, and irregular heartbeat.

Sexual Side Effects of Antidepressant Drugs

With antidepressants, an unfortunate trade-off is sometimes encountered: Some of the drugs that are most effective in relieving depression can adversely affect sexual functioning in both men and women. Common side effects include inhibited arousal and diminished intensity of orgasms. Women may have difficulty becoming lubricated, and men may have trouble getting or maintaining erections and ejaculating.

> **I have suffered from severe depression for years, and recently was given Prozac by a therapist. My mood is better than ever, but I don't feel much interest in sex anymore. It takes forever for me to have an orgasm. My husband has been patient, but we both feel frustrated. What can I do about this?**

You've hit on a true dilemma: There really is no solution short of giving up the medication. Some patients suffering from chronic, disabling depression view the loss of their sexual drive as an acceptable price to pay for treating the depression. One woman I treated who was no longer able to have orgasms after taking medication said her marriage was dramatically improved simply because she was no longer depressed. Sex with her husband was closer and more satisfying, even without orgasm.

Each case is different, and you have to assess what is more important to you at this time—improved mood or your normal sexual functioning. You should discuss the pros and cons of medication with your partner. See your doctor to ask if the medication can be adjusted or changed. I have recommended that my own patients take the medication as prescribed for 6–8 months and then try going off it. If the depression returns, it is always possible to resume the medication.

Chapter 12

AIDS and Sex—What You Don't Know Could Hurt You!

We currently are in the midst of a new sexual revolution, and its catalyst is the heartrending specter of acquired immunodeficiency syndrome (AIDS). The spread of this deadly disease dictates that all of us must constantly reassess our patterns of dating, courtship, living together, marriage, and parenting to ensure that we minimize our chance of contracting and spreading human immunodeficiency virus (HIV), the virus that causes AIDS. Above all, it requires that everyone be more selective and more assertive about their sex lives. Yet this message is difficult to get across.

The epidemic aspects of AIDS, as well as other sexually transmitted diseases (STDs), have forced far more open discussions about sex than were possible before. Schools, doctors, public health organizations, and the media all have been urged to take roles in providing information about how people can incorporate safe sex into their lives.

Despite all the talking and reporting on the dangers of AIDS and its impact on people's lives, however, many movers and shakers in the media—writers, editors, directors, producers, and the like—continue to portray sex as easy, uncomplicated, and unencumbered. People who don't embrace this position may have a sense of isolation and worry that somehow this neorevolution has passed them by.

Movies, television shows, magazines, and books remain dominated by unrealistic portrayals of sex, in which everyone is uninhibited, has beautiful bodies, automatically knows what to do in bed, and experiences no uncertainty or worry. These unrealistic images set the standards by which all too many of us measure ourselves, and they influence behavior, too.

It's my belief that most people want to practice safe sex, but they sometimes engage in unsafe sexual practices because they may be embarrassed to question their partner or may simply throw caution to the wind and operate with the hope that "it won't happen to me." They may not have been taught how to ask questions that revolve around safe sexual practices. People will often tell themselves that AIDS doesn't exist in their crowd or that it doesn't happen to nice people. Only recently, I heard a physician tell a patient not to worry about sex with her new boyfriend because he was a "decent" guy. As if the virus knows the difference!

There is no cure for AIDS, no good treatment to control it, and no vaccine to prevent it. The virus is an equal-opportunity killer that knows no boundaries of age, religion, education, occupation, ethnic group, or social or marital status.

AIDS research still has a long way to go in unraveling the mysteries of HIV. We don't understand why some people contract the virus after one encounter with an infected person while others remain uninfected after many such encounters. People used to reassure themselves with the belief that it was only drug users and homosexuals who were at risk. Now we know that this is simply not true. *Anyone* who is sexually active is at risk. In its semiannual HIV/AIDS Surveillance Report (June 1995), the Centers for Disease Control and Prevention (CDC) reported the cumulative number of reported AIDS cases as 476,899 (405,462 in men, 64,822 in women, and 6,611 in children). The CDC reports that 35,683 of these cases are in individuals identifying themselves as exclusively heterosexual (12,049 men and 23,633 women).

How can a person safely proceed? The answer is more complicated than one might think. Celibacy or abstinence is the only sure route to avoid getting AIDS from sexual encounters, but this is not acceptable to most adults who desire and actively seek sexual expression with another person. Monogamy does not carry an ironclad guarantee. Research shows that many infected women got the virus through sexual contact with an infected partner who they mistakenly thought was faithful. Because the virus may go undetected for years, someone who is monogamous today can still pose a threat to his or her partner because of an exposure several years ago.

Although there are various ways to try to protect yourself from the AIDS virus, sex with an infected person can never be 100% safe. Totally safe sex can take place only with someone who is absolutely knowledgeable and trustworthy when he or she claims to be infection-free. I'm not trying to frighten anyone away from sex. Sexual satisfaction is one of the most important factors for happiness. It is to be shared and enjoyed, not feared and dreaded. Sexuality is not the culprit!

I do believe, however, that unless people accept the danger involved in a sexual encounter, they are unlikely to take control of their sex lives in ways that will substantially reduce their risks.

I am suggesting a healthy skepticism about prospective partners and a slower waltz into the bedroom. Spend more time at the beginning of a relationship in talking, sharing, and other forms of nonphysical intimacy. Opt in the beginning not to engage in sexual intercourse but to focus on activities such as sexually arousing touching, massage, rubbing fully clothed bodies together, mutual masturbation, or sharing erotica. Strive for long-term, committed relationships and learn to derive sexual pleasure from your own body without a partner.

Caution can actually enhance sexual satisfaction. In one study, college students in monogamous relationships had intercourse al-

most twice as many times a year as those in nonexclusive relationships. It is likely that a "committed" couple will develop more trust
and be in a position to learn more about each other's sexual likes
and dislikes, resulting in more rewarding sexual experiences. These
findings have recently been confirmed in the University of Chicago
study "Sex in America" (Laumann, Michael, and Gagnon 1994).

A careful approach to physical relationships in the Age of AIDS
is a matter of life and death; more talk before sex can only add to
a relationship.

Topics covered in this chapter include the following:

* Safer condom use
* Back in the dating scene after 14 years
* AIDS and oral sex
* Safer oral sex
* Boyfriend doesn't want to use condoms

What is the best way to use a condom, and is there any way to increase its effectiveness?

Although condoms are cheap, easy to buy, and help protect against
the spread of the virus that causes AIDS, they are not foolproof.
They must be properly put on and taken off. Like any other manufactured product, condoms are occasionally defective.

Here is a 10-step guide to safer condom use:

1. Buy only latex condoms. Condoms made of animal skins are
   for contraceptive use only. They do not protect against AIDS
   or other STDs.
2. Properly stored, a condom will be usable for several years. Do
   not keep a condom in your wallet where it may get bent and
   split and where it will be exposed to body heat, which can
   cause deterioration.
3. Choose condoms with receptacle tips to catch ejaculate. Also,
   buy ones that are lubricated with the spermicide nonoxynol-9,
   at least 5%, and check the expiration date. Spermicide pro-

vides extra protection from pregnancy and STDs should the condom leak. *Note:* Some people are allergic to spermicide. There are alternatives, including Erogel, a product made of nonoxynol-15, manufactured by the Institute for Advanced Study of Human Sexuality. As for size, bigger is not better. It's a rare man who needs an extra-large condom. Using one just increases the danger of the condom coming off during intercourse.

4. Do not use condoms with oil-based vaginal or anal lubricants, such as Vaseline, baby oil, Crisco, or vegetable oil. Oil will melt the latex, creating minute holes and eventually causing breakage. Water-soluble lubricants, such as K-Y Jelly, saliva, or plain tap water, are okay. Note, too, that oil-based foods or animal fats will degrade the latex, so do not use whipped cream or ice cream with a condom. Water-based substances are okay, including honey, wine, or champagne.

5. Open the condom package carefully, being cautious not to rip the latex with your fingernails. Before unrolling it, put a tiny drop of spermicide in the tip, if available.

6. Place the still-rolled condom onto the tip of the penis and slowly unroll it all the way to the base of the penis. Gently smooth out any air bubbles. If two men are having sex together, both should wear condoms.

7. Never insert the penis into a partner's body any farther than the condom reaches, or it could slip off.

8. Withdraw the penis soon after ejaculation, holding onto the condom around the base of the penis to make sure that it does not come off.

9. The man should remove the condom himself. This will prevent his partner from coming in direct contact with semen. Do not allow your sex organs to touch after the condom has been removed.

10. Never use a condom more than once.

Note: For added protection against leakage, a woman can use a diaphragm coated with nonoxynol-9 while the man wears a con-

dom. Another option is to use a female condom made of polyure-
thane, which is inserted into the vagina.

> **I am 35 years old and recently got divorced after 14 years of
> marriage. To be honest, I feel like a teenager again when I
> think of dating and getting into a sexual relationship. I have
> no idea how to talk to potential partners about AIDS. What
> would you advise?**

Talking about sensitive issues is easier once you get to know a potential partner. Delaying decisions about becoming sexual until
you know the person better will make the discussion more comfortable. We are gradually emerging from decades of viewing sex
as an easy and quick way to get to know someone. Today, that
attitude is not only frivolous but dangerous. In reality, it never was
a good idea and often made relationships feel serious and committed without any of the deep emotional attachments needed to
make such feelings real.

Having a sense of who another person is—what he or she likes
and dislikes, the values you share, and how it feels to spend time
together—helps form bonds that provide a foundation for a long-
term relationship. By waiting, you will have the opportunity to
explore dimensions of the relationship that will be enhanced when
you finally become sexual.

You will have to learn how to have open, frank discussions with
potential partners about previous sexual relationships. Of course,
this is a difficult, sensitive, and embarrassing task to take on. In the
past, people struggled with their sexual insecurities and feeling
incompetent, with few words spoken to make the passage
smoother. Now the pressure is really on to ask explicit questions.
It is sometimes helpful to practice asking questions, either alone
(perhaps speaking to a tape recorder) or with a good friend. The
more you practice, the more comfortable you will be when you
have to bring up the topic.

An opener can be, "I've really enjoyed getting to know you and
would like our relationship to grow. We need to talk about a sensitive

topic: other sexual relationships we've each had. I hope we can discuss what our patterns have been and whether we have been at risk for exposure to AIDS."

If you can't bring yourself to bring up the topic, try steering a conversation in that direction by saying something like, "I love watching soap operas. But I can't believe how everyone is still flying in and out of each other's bedrooms. I'd be too scared, with all the sexually transmitted diseases out there. Do you agree?"

Before you engage in any sexual activity, you'll want to know that your partner is free of the AIDS virus. Unless he was recently tested and shares that information, clues will have to come from answers to questions such as these:

* How many sex partners have you had in the last 7 years?
* Have you had sex with a gay or bisexual man in that time?
* Have you recently had a blood transfusion or slept with some- one who did?
* Do you or did you ever do intravenous drugs?
* Did you ever have intercourse with an intravenous drug user?

Short of hiring a private detective, you'll have to rely on your own intuition to tell you if your partner is being truthful.

Finally, be sure to ask these two questions:

* What safer sex techniques do you most enjoy?
* Are you willing to be tested?

Can you catch AIDS from oral sex?

The AIDS virus can be found in an infected man's ejaculate or in an infected woman's vaginal secretions. Therefore, if a man's pree-jaculatory fluid or semen enters his partner's mouth and the part-ner has any cuts or mouth sores, it is possible that HIV could enter the bloodstream. Similarly, a man or woman who has sores in the mouth risks being infected by vaginal secretions if he or she per-forms oral sex.

Although a very high percentage of couples (between 80% and 90%) engage in oral sex at some time, the Centers for Disease Control and Prevention has yet to document any cases in which HIV was transmitted during oral sex. However, it is important to stress that we don't have all the answers, and in this case, I would advocate caution. The virus is found in semen and in vaginal secretions; the gums and lining of the mouth can easily be traumatized and could theoretically provide a passage for the virus.

So, how do you make oral sex safe?

You should perform fellatio (a "blow job") only when a man is wearing a latex condom over his penis. Manufacturers of condoms have been quick to respond by creating mint-flavored condoms that don't taste like latex. Otherwise, it helps to gently wipe the condom with plain water before putting it in your mouth.

Never agree to unprotected oral sex because a man promises not to come in your mouth. Studies show that 75% of men secrete preejaculatory fluid that may contain HIV if the man is infected.

Safe cunnilingus (kissing or licking the vagina) requires using a dental dam, a 6-inch square made of latex, the same material as condoms. The dam is stretched over the vulva, including the clitoris, lips, and vagina. Oral stimulation—tonguing, sucking, licking—is done through the latex barrier. Dental dams also are used to cover the anus for oral-anal stimulation. They usually are sold alongside condoms.

Remember: What little sensation you lose by using a barrier is more than made up by the comfort of knowing you are protecting yourself or your partner from a fatal disease.

I am very concerned about AIDS and protecting myself. However, my boyfriend is uncomfortable about using condoms and says he does not want to. What should I do?

First, I commend taking responsibility for your health. AIDS is a matter of life and death, and everyone needs to be aware of what they can do to make sure that sex is safer. You did not say why your boyfriend will not use condoms, so let me raise some of the more common arguments:

* *I am too embarrassed to buy them.* At one time, condoms were sold only by druggists and usually stored behind the counter. It was awkward to ask for them, doubly so when the druggist might ask what size you wanted. Those days are long gone. Today, condoms are sold openly in supermarkets, drugstores, newsstands, rest rooms, and chain stores. Most major cities have at least one specialty condom shop that stocks prophylactics from around the world. There are many mail-order companies that will wrap condoms in plain paper and deliver them right to your door.

* *They interfere with spontaneity.* If you keep condoms close at hand, there's no reason for spontaneity to be reduced. Imaginative couples easily can make condom use part of lovemaking. Many people find that sensuously putting on a condom can turn a soft penis hard in a matter of seconds. Having a man sheathed as soon as he has an erection also eliminates any reason to stop for a moment when things heat up.

* *They take away from sensation.* Initially, this may be true. But most men find that as the condom warms to body temperature, the barrier to sensation diminishes. The variety of latex condoms is vast, so shop around if you don't like the feel of one brand. Try lubricated, formfitting, textured, and thin-skinned types. You and your boyfriend should find one that is right for both of you.*

**Men's Health* magazine reviewed condoms in an article titled "What to Wear in Bed" in its July/August 1994 issue. One condom stood out as rating an "A+" for sensitivity—Pleasure Plus by Reddy Labs. The condom is snug at the bottom, with plenty of room at the top. The review claimed that "it was the next best thing to skin on skin—for me *and* my partner" (Roman 1994, p. 40).

If he continues to refuse, you could simply say, "I like being with you, but I can't relax and get turned on if you don't use a condom."

A final observation: Perhaps your boyfriend's refusal to wear a condom will be a catalyst to reexamining the relationship. After all, a man who refuses to use a condom—thus minimizing his partner's concerns—is telling her that her needs will not be taken seriously in this relationship. His reaction may tell you that you have no real future together.

Chapter 13

Variations, or "Why Don't They Teach That in Sex Ed?"

Sitting in my office listening to the stories of people's lives, I am constantly struck by the almost limitless variations of interests and activities for people, and nowhere is this more the case than in their sexual interests and choices. It is one thing to read about "bondage" in a book and quite another to have people tell you about their experiences and try to explain why it turns them on. The more researchers ask people what they do, the more information we have about trends and patterns of behavior. Although the behaviors on the "fringe" might get a lot of publicity, most people are still fairly conventional when it comes to their sexual interests. Still, many are curious about variations and need some information to make informed decisions.

Topics covered in this chapter include the following:

* Anal sex
* Body piercing

* Bondage
* Rough sex
* When a raincoat is all I wear
* Sex in public
* Swapping
* S&M (sadomasochism)
* Fetish for underwear
* I'm dating a nudist
* Perversion
* Aphrodisiacs
* Vibrators

My boyfriend likes to have anal sex. I've tried it but usually bleed slightly afterward. Should I be concerned? Will it lead to rectal cancer?

Anal sex is much more a part of couples' repertoire than people realize. Depending on the study being cited, between 20% and 40% of married women report having tried anal sex at least once. This activity will *not* lead to rectal cancer. There are a few guidelines, though:

1. Use a lubricant (such as Astroglide or K-Y Jelly) and make sure your partner is gentle. This probably will help reduce your bleeding.
2. If neither partner is infected, anal sex does not cause AIDS. If one partner is infected, however, the risk of transmitting the virus is high, probably because the rectal tissues are easily damaged during intercourse. Use a condom unless you are absolutely sure your partner is infection-free.
3. After anal intercourse, your partner must thoroughly wash his penis before you take it into your vagina or mouth. Bacteria from the rectum can lead to serious medical problems if introduced into the vagina through intercourse.
4. As always, this is an activity in which it is important that both are willing participants.

My girlfriend has been talking about body piercing lately. It intrigues me. What do you think?

Body piercing involves puncturing unconventional sites, including nose, nipples, belly button, labia, clitoris, and penis, and inserting metal rings, sometimes with jewelry attached, through the holes.

I realize that the freedom to do what we please is precious, but to me body piercing is carrying things to a bizarre extreme. Some forms of body piercing may not cause physical harm, but I believe that the practice itself reflects some strange wishes. For example, I've heard of people who have had their nipples pierced with rings that had chains attached to them, so partners could restrain them and inflict pain. The point of all this is to give the aggressor a sense of power over the other person. This, I believe, is quite a distortion of the normal give-and-take of relationships.

Most people who engage in body piercing will deny that there is anything abnormal about it. For some, it may be their current fashion statement and declaration of independence. However, when it is more than just a passing interest, I believe that something more destructive is being expressed.

My husband and I have been married for 5 years. Recently he has begun talking more about doing things sexually that I think are kinky. He would like to try spanking and some "light bondage" with handcuffs. The whole idea gives me the creeps. I thought that I was open-minded, but this really turns me off. Still, I'm afraid that if I don't comply, he will search elsewhere for satisfaction.

Every couple should be guided by a respect and reverence for each other's feelings. The *only* acceptable activities in any particular relationship are ones that *both* partners are comfortable with. Sexuality is a means for expressing very powerful feelings between two people, and open communication, comfort, and respect really make a difference. Ask your husband to tell you more about what exactly he has in mind and how he came up with this idea. If you do not want to do what he asks, tell him so directly.

However, if your husband persists in wanting you to act on his ideas and you continue to worry about consequences if you don't acquiesce, talking with a neutral third party such as a counselor would be useful. It may help to understand the meaning behind his requests and to clarify to him your unwillingness to be coerced. Sometimes, once people get closer to the reality of an expressed wish or fantasy, the idea seems less appealing.

> **My husband and I love each other very much. However, he likes quick, rough sex in which he dominates and leads, but this gives me little satisfaction. I want to spend time kissing, holding, and touching, but he does not enjoy these. I've told him my feelings, and now we have no sex at all. What do we do now?**

You have reinforced the point I made in the previous question. If one partner does not enjoy a particular activity, sex is not going to be satisfying. What you describe is your husband's need to do it his way, with very little regard for what you enjoy. In other words, sex becomes a vehicle for his expressing domination and power, and shared closeness is not possible. I would suggest talking with a counselor; this would provide a forum to try to understand your differences and see if it is possible for your husband to find pleasure in a more mutual sexual expression.

> **I've been seeing this guy on and off for 5 years. The problem is that when we have sex, I like it rough. He doesn't. But what if I like the pain? Is there something wrong with me?**

It sounds as if you and the previous writer have gotten your partners mixed up! It seems as if sex has become a vehicle for you to receive pain and be treated badly. I wonder why you need to seek out this kind of treatment. You seem a little uncomfortable about whether this feeling is okay, and a counselor might help you sort it out. There are a few things to consider:

* Do you have any recollection of any verbal, physical, or sexual abuse as a child?
* Was there any history of alcoholism in your family? In 65% of families where the father is alcoholic, there is physical or sexual abuse.
* Do you struggle with feelings of low self-esteem? You may express this by allowing other people to treat you badly.

> I love to walk down the street wearing nothing but an unbuttoned raincoat. My boyfriend loves to stand on a corner and watch the expressions of passersby who get to glimpse my nakedness. Is there anything wrong with doing this?

Although there's no question that experimentation can provide excitement and new experiences, some sexual activities are "atypical" and appeal to fewer people. These include exhibitionism (the wish to be sexual in public) and voyeurism (the wish to watch). These activities generally are harmless to consenting adults who engage in them but may be traumatic to any person who is drawn in as an unsuspecting party. For some exhibitionists, part of the thrill and excitement is derived from shocking others with their behavior. Apart from the fact that "flashing" is illegal, the consequences for "victims" can be painful and unwelcome.

> Is it weird to have sex in public places? One of my many fantasies is about having a "quickie" with my husband in an elevator between floors.

It can be very exciting to do things you consider "naughty"—acts that in some way challenge authority or test boundaries. In most cases, this instinct is natural and harmless, and it can be a refreshing variation in a couple's routine. It's the desire for change or newness that is most likely behind your fantasy. The spontaneity of having sex in a strange place turns you on, and if you use good judgment, acting on this should not offend anyone.

On the other hand, when the intention is simply to expose what you do sexually with your husband to others, it crosses over into the realm of exhibitionism, which is a psychological problem. In this instance, the intent is to foist upon an unsuspecting audience actions that are traditionally personal and private. It is offensive to many of the people who might unwittingly have to witness it and is disrespectful of their privacy.

Only you know your intentions. If they're innocent, you may want to choose some place more discreet than an elevator to act on them—maybe a private picnic in the woods? But if you fear that your fantasy stems from an unhealthy urge, you should probably rethink it.

> **I recently read an article by a couple who said swapping partners with other couples added excitement to their marriage. My husband and I have talked about doing this. Is it dangerous?**

"Swinging" became popular in the 1960s, when a dramatic change occurred in the social norms regarding sexuality. Many Americans went from a fairly conservative attitude about sex to an "anything goes" philosophy.

Several social scientists have speculated that the sexual revolution was created by the concurrent development of the pill, the rise of the women's liberation movement, and protests against the Vietnam War, in which defiance of authority was so prominent.

Swinging clubs where people can meet one another and make appointments still exist, and it's not unusual to find couples advertising for other couples in the personal ads. Once they get together, a leader may organize what people do and with whom, or it may be more of a free-for-all format.

Swinging is not for everyone. The first concern is AIDS and other STDs. The risk of contracting any STD increases dramatically as you increase your number of sexual partners. So if you do choose to participate, you should use extreme caution.

Another concern is unanticipated feelings of jealousy. People may think that the idea of their partner having sex with someone else will not threaten them, but the reality may be very different. The situation may also challenge your or your partner's self-esteem and cause feelings of insecurity. I believe there are alternative ways to add spark to your relationship that would entail fewer risks.

You need to think of this like opening Pandora's box—you don't know what you might unleash, and the consequences may not be good. Many who have engaged in swapping describe their experiences in positive terms; they are unlikely to seek therapy, as the behavior has not been perceived as problematic. The couples I have usually seen are those like you, in which one partner is interested and the other unwilling. Almost invariably, the marriage has been on a shaky footing, and the discussion about swinging reflected other problems.

> **I found a disturbing book at a friend's house, all about getting aroused while beating and whipping other people. Frankly, I was shocked. Who would want to read such a thing?**

What you are describing is a book about sadism. (*The Story of O* is one well-known book dealing with extreme forms of sadistic behavior.) In sadism, a person gets sexual pleasure by inflicting pain on another person. The other side of that particular coin is masochism, where sexual pleasure comes from receiving physical pain. The ways these activities are performed vary from very mild, where people act out a situation but do not inflict harm, to perverse forms of sexual attack and violence that include rape or unwilling bondage or, in extreme forms, murder.

Sadomasochism is part of a whole group of behaviors called *paraphilias* because they are outside social norms. According to the Kinsey Institute, approximately 5% to 10% of the United States population engage in sadomasochism for sexual pleasure on at least an occasional basis.

While consenting adults may try these behaviors, in anything but the mildest forms they represent serious distortions of interpersonal relationships. People who feel compelled to participate in sadomasochistic sex often come from dysfunctional families. As children, they may have felt powerless against physical abuse or severe emotional deprivation. In ways we don't entirely understand, their pain is linked with sexual arousal. As adults, they may wish to inflict pain on another individual, and the sexual arena becomes the place in which to play out this desire. Most people do not "choose" to be turned on by this behavior, though many who are attracted to it can satisfy their curiosity without action. Instead, they read books such as the one you describe.

A new form of this activity has developed on the on-line computer services and even has a name—"cybersex." There are forums and bulletin boards where people talk about their wishes to dominate others in relationships or to be submissive (called *domming* and *subbing*). The descriptions are quite graphic and involve discussions of elaborate accessories, including whips, chains, and other instruments for afflicting pain. I have tried to understand this behavior, but I can only think of it as reflecting serious disturbances relating to very early childhood experiences. I cannot accept sadomasochistic behavior as a "normal" variant. For many who engage in this behavior, though, there is no sense of angst about their activities. Although it is getting more media attention recently, I see no reason to view this as possible "mainstream" behavior.

> **When women wear lacy panty hose I go wild. My friends tease me that I've got a fetish. What exactly is a fetish?**

The dictionary meaning of the word fetish is "an object that has magical or spiritual powers." In sexual terms, an individual has a fetish when he or she is so turned on by an object that it replaces the person as a source of sexual gratification. (Fetishes have been studied mostly in men.)

You seem worried that you especially like to see women's legs covered in a particular way. It sounds as if that's just something that is attractive to you. You might have a fetish, however, if simply holding a pair of lacy panty hose in your hands got you aroused or if you paid more attention to the panty hose than your partner during lovemaking.

> I am dating a man who is a nudist. He wants me not to wear clothes around his apartment and to go to a nude beach. I think the idea is weird, but I'd like to be open-minded. Any suggestions?

We could learn something from the Europeans when it comes to this issue. My sense is that Europeans tend to be more open and comfortable with their bodies than most Americans; we seem to be burdened with a heightened sense of modesty and spend more time and effort trying to "whip our bodies into shape" rather than seeing them as sources of pleasure and enjoyment. Most likely, the man you are dating has a healthy sense of comfort about his body and welcomes the freedom of being unencumbered by clothing.

If you can look on this as an adventure and a chance to open yourself to new experiences, certainly try the nudist lifestyle. If, on the other hand, you dread the experience and know you won't be able to overcome your initial embarrassment, I suggest you pass on the adventure.

> If you imagine a situation, but don't try it—such as having sex with animals or wanting to be treated like a slave—are you a pervert?

Let's try to understand first what we mean by the term *pervert*. In psychiatric terms, it refers to a process in which the emotional energy usually directed to an individual is transferred to a very different direction, perverting the original intent. For example, in having sex with an animal, the original impulse, to be close and intimate with another human being, is transformed and "perverted" in a different direction.

Having said that, let me add that there are different degrees to which an individual may be preoccupied and affected by a perversion of interest. It may be confined to imagining what most people would term "unnatural acts" and feeling some sexual arousal in the process, or it might include trying to perform or succeeding in performing a particular act. Perversions include a wide range of activities such as sex with animals, eating feces, and a variety of forms of dismembering.

A friend of mine told me of a news report about a special drug to increase your sex drive. He also swears that marijuana makes him enjoy sex more intensely. Could these be true aphrodisiacs?

Throughout time, people have been searching for substances that enhance sexual prowess. Overall, the results have been disappointing. Like your friend, some people who smoke marijuana say it gives them an enhanced awareness and sensitivity to touch that makes sex better. But the aphrodisiac effects of marijuana and other street drugs are variable, and all lead to inhibited sexual desire with constant use. Many people also mistakenly believe that alcohol facilitates sex because it lowers inhibitions. However, in several studies, even small amounts of alcohol were shown to depress sexual responsiveness and ability. Cocaine is another drug that's been touted as offering sexual power. In truth, it very often leads to sexual dysfunction.

Since you're asking about increasing desire, it's possible that either you or your partner has experienced a dramatic decrease in sex drive. If that is so, you should consult a physician to rule out depression, a hormonal or thyroid problem, or other conditions that can decrease sexual functioning.

The search for aphrodisiacs, however, is worldwide. Yohimbine (an extract from a tree found in Africa), which folk healers have used to treat erectile difficulties and low libido, has not yielded impressive results. The myth that rhino horn has mystical properties that affect sex drive has probably contributed more to the decline of that species than to anyone's pleasure.

In short, there is no miracle drug, legal or otherwise, that will reliably increase sexual desire. Researchers continue their attempts to understand the biochemistry of sexual drive, and who knows, perhaps one day they will. The most promising things on the horizon are pheromones—substances secreted by animals to attract members of the opposite sex through their sense of smell. Farmers already can buy synthetic insect pheromones to help control infestation of their crops. Work on human pheromones is still in its infancy, however.

A friend of mine raves about using a vibrator during sex. I'm curious but afraid. Are vibrators unnatural or deviant?

There's nothing new about people trying to enhance their sexual pleasure with devices—they've been doing so throughout history. Modern technology has taken a quantum leap, allowing the creation of a dazzling display of "accessories" limited only by the imagination. Whether their claims are overrated is for the individual consumer to decide. Some find that these devices are as indispensable as a hair dryer, while many others find that they become a mechanical distraction. Today, you can easily buy a vibrator from any department store or large drugstore. These electric massagers come in two basic forms. One is electrically operated, hand-held, and comes with different adapters that fit over the vibrating end. They are advertised as providing relief to aching muscles, but they are often used for sexual stimulation. The adapters, which may be shaped like a cup, a fingertip, or a circle of rubber tips, offer variations in intensity. These kinds of vibrators are recommended by sex therapists to help women who have trouble reaching orgasm. (Explicit techniques are described in a book-and-video set called *Becoming Orgasmic*. See the appendix ["Information Resources"] at the end of this book.)

The second type of vibrator is a battery-operated cylinder shaped more like a penis. These can be inserted into the vagina and are obviously designed for sexual purposes. They come in a variety of dimensions and colors; I suspect the variety is chiefly a marketing ploy. As with any sexual issue, certain rules apply: If you are comfortable, trusting of your partner, and engaged in a mutually agreeable activity, try it and see if it does anything for you. You may have to try it a few times to get over the initial reaction that it feels like "robo sex," but collect your own data and make your decision.

One word of caution: The anus is richly supplied with nerves, which is why touching it is an enjoyable part of lovemaking for many couples. Sometimes people find it pleasurable to insert small vibrators into the anus. Hygiene, however, is crucial. Never place a vibrator that has been used for anal stimulation in the vagina until it has been washed thoroughly. Gentleness and lubrication are key, and if you experience pain, don't continue using it.

If you find that using a vibrator to stimulate each other's genitals gives you both feelings of pleasure and provides a different kind of intense arousal, keep it at the bedside. However, if it feels mechanical and impersonal to you, forget it. Many couples who have tried vibrators decide the devices are not a turn-on.

A _ppendix_

Information Resources

Books

Ask Me Anything: A Sex Therapist Answers the Most Important Questions for the '90s. Marty Klein, Ph.D. New York, Simon & Schuster, 1992.
The format of this book is question and answer. It's like having a conversation with a benevolent uncle who enjoys talking with you, is direct, and has much to offer.

Becoming Orgasmic. Julia R. Heiman, Ph.D., and Joseph LoPiccolo, Ph.D. New York, Prentice-Hall, 1988.
This book, in conjunction with the tape produced by FOCUS INTERNATIONAL, is a great resource. It educates by discussing anatomy and physiological responses, and it deals specifically with the way people become blocked sexually. The authors are extremely experienced and give specific suggestions and exercises to help women. The tape, I believe, is essential to complement the text: The "thoughts" you hear of the subject's concerns in the tape resonate with what I so frequently hear in my office. It is also a book that many men should read.

ESO [Extended Sexual Orgasm] Alan P. Brauer, Donna Brauer, and Richard Rhodes. New York, Warner Books, 1989.
Although the emphasis in the title ("Extended Sexual Orgasm") appears to be on Olympic training, the book has good suggestions in the section dealing with premature ejaculation.

The Family Book About Sexuality. Mary S. Calderone, M.D., and Eric W. Johnson. New York, Harper & Row, 1989.
For parents who need guidance in what kids need to know and how to talk about it, this book is clearly written, encouraging, and comprehensive. Almost all the patients I see who struggle with sexuality had virtually no information or guidance from their parents. We are eager and encouraging when it comes to instruction for everything else from piano lessons to driving, but sex is somehow off limits. There are cultures where children are instructed and taught about their bodies and about sexual practices, and I believe we have much to learn from that approach. This book provides a framework for discussion with your children.

Female Sexual Awareness: Achieving Sexual Fulfillment. Barry McCarthy and Emily McCarthy. New York, Carroll & Graf, 1989.
Male Sexual Awareness: Increasing Sexual Pleasure. Barry McCarthy. New York, Carroll & Graf, 1988.
These two books follow a traditional approach; they contain much information and are oriented for readers who are interested in theory and therapy.

The Good Vibrations Guide to Sex: How to Have Safe, Fun Sex in the 90s. Cathy Winks and Anne Semans. San Francisco, CA, Cleis Press, 1994.
This is a thorough, well-written, and well-researched book that covers the field comprehensively. The writing is clear and informative, and avoids gender biases and value judgments. The authors provide information that is generally not well done in many other books: topics include "All About Vibrators"; "All About Dildos";

"All About Anal Toys"; "Books, Magazines, and Videos"; and "S&M and Power Play." In addition, they have a number of helpful, practical suggestions that are presented in a direct, playful way.

Hot, Sexy and Safer. Suzi Landolphi. New York, Berkeley Publishing Group, 1994.

Suzi Landolphi is the cofounder of Condomania, a company pioneering a new way to market condoms. This is a great, no-nonsense book that is particularly good for teenage girls in terms of promoting good "sexual self-esteem." Teenage boys will also benefit from learning more about the sexual responses of women, and with a great deal of humor be exposed to some of the sillier gender stereotypes. For those of us adults who had no wonderful Aunt Fannie or Uncle Max when we were growing up, the book is fun to read and helpful in provoking thinking about what we would like our kids to learn.

The Illustrated Manual of Sex Therapy, 2nd Edition. Helen Singer Kaplan. New York, Brunner/Mazel, 1987.

Although now a little dated, this book was the first to provide good illustrations to complement the "exercises" assigned to help couples with sexual difficulties.

The Kinsey Institute New Report on Sex. June M. Reinisch, Ph.D., and Ruth Beasley, M.L.S. New York, St. Martin's Press, 1991.

Kinsey was the first researcher to collect data on the sexual practices of American men and women. He broke the silence by asking people what they did and then published the results. The Kinsey Institute book is in question-and-answer format; it covers everything you could ever want to know about sexuality, including development, dysfunctions and treatment, abuse, and sexually transmitted diseases. It has extensive reading lists and resources for a variety of different services. It might be the kind of book you would take out of the library rather than buy. It is impressively thorough and inclusive.

Masters and Johnson on Sex and Human Loving. William H. Masters, M.D., Virginia E. Johnson, Ph.D., and Robert C. Kolodny, M.D. Boston, MA, Little, Brown, 1988.
This is a comprehensive textbook written by well-known people; the information is extensive and thorough. I have found it very helpful when I need to get specific information. It is written in a straightforward manner.

The New Male Sexuality. Bernie Zilbergeld, Ph.D. New York, Bantam Books, 1992.
Bernie Zilbergeld is a psychologist on the West Coast who has worked extensively with individuals and couples on sexuality. The title of this book does not do justice to its broad scope. He describes male psychological development with clarity and humor. He prefaces his discussion by elaborating on the progress that has been made over the years in understanding female development, but he points out that there has been a silent assumption that we know what is involved for men. He feels the need for a parallel exposition regarding the developmental and interpersonal needs of men, and he does a remarkably good job of providing it. He integrates this with an understanding of sexual physiology for men, details concerns and worries, dispels many myths, and writes impressively about the travails of being a couple. This book is well written, clear, and extremely useful for both men and women.

The New Our Bodies, Ourselves: A Book by and for Women. Boston Women's Collective. New York, Simon & Schuster, 1992.
Anyone who grew up in the 1960s will remember the original edition of this homegrown book. Written by women who realized every woman's need for good, reliable information about her body, the book has expanded over the years to include much helpful advice regarding sexuality, gender issues, and many other timely topics.

The Potent Male: Facts, Fiction, Future. Irwin Goldstein, M.D., and Larry Rothstein. Los Angeles, CA, Body Press, 1990.
I wish this book had been available many years ago. It is an excel-

lent review of male dysfunctions; what is truly unique is that it includes medical, surgical, and psychological factors. The authors have produced a comprehensive text filled with informative diagrams and tables, and the accounts written by Dr. Goldstein's patients are an invaluable addition. I would strongly recommend this book for any couple with erectile difficulties. Being informed and educated helps people be effective advocates in their treatment.

The Sex Encyclopedia. Prevention **magazine editors and Stefan Bechtel. New York, Simon & Schuster, 1993.**
Arranged in alphabetical order, the entries in this book give current information about the whole range of sexual behavior. The book is easy to read and good to have around as a resource.

Sexual Happiness: A Practical Approach. **Maurice Yaffe and Elizabeth Fenwick. New York, Henry Holt, 1988.**
This team obviously wrote this book when computer graphics were becoming popular. The diagrams and flowcharts are truly dazzling. The book has great illustrations, particularly for sexual positions. There are sections with specific self-help approaches that are basically sound.

The Ultimate Sex Book. **Anne Hooper. New York, Dorling Kindersley, 1992.**
Topics covered include erotica, gay/lesbian issues, female issues, male issues, menopause, safer sex, sex and aging, sex education for kids, sexual enhancement, and sexual self-help.

Teaching and Self-Help Videos

FOCUS INTERNATIONAL, based in New York, has been producing and distributing videotapes dealing with sexuality for nearly 20 years. The tapes are well done, instructive, and graphic. The information is current, and having couples demonstrate the techniques adds to their effectiveness. Call 1-800-843-0305 to receive a catalog, or visit it on the Internet at http://www/hip.com/focus. The following videos are recommended:

* *Becoming Orgasmic.* Julia R. Heiman, Ph.D., and Joseph LoPiccolo, Ph.D.
* *Sexual Positions—Beyond the Missionary Position.* Derek Polonsky, M.D., and Marian Dunn, Ph.D.
* *Treating Erectile Difficulties.* Joseph LoPiccolo, Ph.D.
* *Treating Vaginismus.* Joseph LoPiccolo, Ph.D.
* *You Can Last Longer.* Derek Polonsky, M.D., and Marian Dunn, Ph.D.

Vacuum Pumps for Erectile Difficulties

ErecAid System, Osbon Medical Systems, P.O. Drawer 1408, Augusta, GA 30903-9990

Vacuum Erection Device, Mission Pharmacy Company, P.O. Box 1676, San Antonio, TX 78296

Post T Vac, P.O. Box 1436, Dodge City, KS 67801

Synergist Ltd., 6910 Fannin, Suite 100, Houston, TX 77030

Vaginal Dilators for Treating Vaginismus

F. E. Young and Company, 1350 Old Skokie Road, Highland Park, IL 60035

Index